THE ILLUSION OF CARE

THE ILLUSION OF CARE

WHY PATIENTS LEAVE CONFUSED AND THE CLINICAL OPERATING SYSTEM THAT FIXES IT

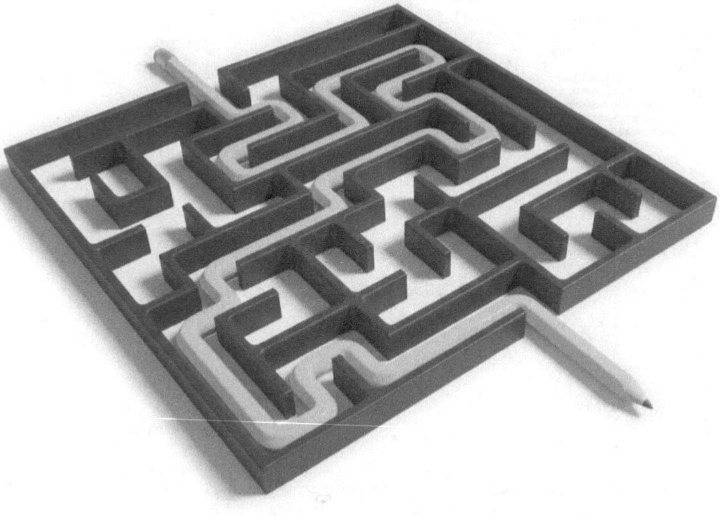

JOSEPH A. ROTELLA, MD, DC

SCRIBE
MEDIA

THE ILLUSION OF CARE
Why Patients Leave Confused and the Clinical Operating System That Fixes It

FIRST EDITION

ISBN 978-1-5445-5404-4 *Hardcover*
978-1-5445-5403-7 *Paperback*
978-1-5445-5405-1 *Ebook*

This book is dedicated to every patient who has ever left a healthcare visit confused, overwhelmed, or uncertain about what to do next.

And to every physician and healthcare professional who believes that care is not complete until every patient truly understands what to do next.

CONTENTS

INTRODUCTION

MEDICINE AT A CROSSROADS

Medicine has changed dramatically over the course of my career. When I first began practicing, healthcare already demanded an extraordinary amount of technical knowledge and clinical precision. But over the years, those demands have only continued to grow, as advances in diagnostics, pharmaceuticals, treatment protocols, and medical technology have transformed what physicians are capable of doing for patients.

In many ways, modern medicine has become extraordinarily effective at identifying disease and managing complex conditions to deliver increasingly sophisticated care. However, at the same time, I have personally witnessed a troubling change, something far less visible but equally important.

The experience of being a patient has become increasingly complicated.

As physicians, we always work hard to make the right diagnosis and choose the best treatment plan because we want to provide the highest quality care possible to every person who comes through the door. We devote years of our lives to learning how to solve extraordinarily complex medical problems, and we bear the burden of that responsibility every single day of our professional lives. Yet after spending decades caring for patients, I noticed a frustrating pattern that seemed to repeat itself over and over again.

All too often, excellent medical care doesn't translate into excellent outcomes, despite our best efforts.

The issue isn't poor medicine or a lack of effort from physicians. It isn't a failure of the healthcare system itself. Instead, I began to recognize a problem hiding behind countless patient interactions, a problem so common that many of us barely stop to question it.

You see, patients frequently leave healthcare meetings without feeling confident about how to implement their care once the visit is over.

This is a big problem because so much of medicine depends on what happens after the appointment is over. The long-term success of almost every treatment plan ultimately depends on a patient's ability to understand what they've been told and remember what actions need to happen next so they can consistently apply those decisions in their everyday life.

Ironically, somewhere along the way, healthcare systems began placing less emphasis on that part of medicine. It wasn't done maliciously. It's something that happened as an unintended consequence of increasing demands in other areas of healthcare.

I experienced this tension firsthand throughout my own career. Like many physicians, I entered medicine because I genuinely wanted to help people improve their health and live better lives. But as the operational demands surrounding healthcare became increasingly complex, I watched the structure of medicine slowly change.

Documentation requirements grew heavier and more elaborate, and schedules became tighter. Administrative responsibilities expanded, and physicians gradually found themselves trying to handle more demands while spending less time focused on one of the most important parts of healthcare: helping patients fully comprehend their health and empowering them to make informed decisions so they could actively participate in their own care.

This communication gap creates consequences far larger than most people realize. When patient understanding breaks down, people struggle to follow treatment plans consistently. Physicians find themselves repeating the same conversations over and over again. Small misunderstandings turn into larger health challenges, and both patients and providers experience growing frustration.

The more I observed this pattern, the more convinced I became that medicine was overlooking an enormous opportunity. What if one of healthcare's greatest opportunities for improvement has less to do with discovering better treatments and more to do with ensuring every patient leaves knowing exactly what to do next?

That question lingered in my mind for years without a clear solution. Eventually, it led me to begin developing my own framework built around the idea that patients need a clear, structured way to know exactly what is happening to them and what actions they need to take, with clear steps they can follow to successfully carry out their care once they return home and begin managing their health on their own.

That framework eventually became something I now call PENCIL. This book tells the story of how that idea developed and why communication may be one of the most overlooked variables affecting healthcare outcomes today. More importantly, I want to show you how physicians can begin approaching patient education in an entirely different and more effective way without adding more complexity to an already demanding profession.

I believe medicine stands at an important crossroads. The future of healthcare will certainly continue to bring better treatments, but some of the most meaningful improvements in patient outcomes may come from transforming patient education into a clear, actionable care plan.

The pages ahead explore why that matters so deeply and why I believe restoring this overlooked part of medicine could fundamentally change how healthcare is delivered for generations to come.

As it turns out, sometimes the most powerful breakthrough is rediscovering something important that was lost along the way.

PART 1

THE FORGOTTEN FOUNDATION OF MEDICINE

CHAPTER 1

WHEN MEDICINE FORGOT TO TEACH

"Doctors once taught as much as they treated. The future of medicine may require both again."

A patient sits across from you in the exam room, listening carefully as you walk through what the last several days or weeks have revealed. You explain the symptoms they're dealing with and connect them to the lab work sitting in front of you. You translate all of the complicated medical terminology into everyday language they can comprehend. You point to numbers on the report, explain what is normal and what is not, and help them understand exactly what is happening inside their body.

Then you begin outlining their treatment plan. You explain the prescription you're recommending and why it's important. You describe when it should be taken, what side effects to watch for, what changes in routine might be necessary to support recovery. You discuss follow-up appointments, lifestyle adjustments, warning signs to monitor, and what success should hopefully look like over the coming weeks.

Throughout the conversation, the patient seems fully engaged. They are looking at you, nodding along as you speak, even offering the occasional acknowledgment. Once you finish, you pause for a moment, giving them time to process everything you've just covered. Then you ask the question every healthcare provider has asked thousands of times before.

"Does all of that make sense?"

For a brief second, there's silence. The patient stares back at you with that familiar expression physicians know all too well. You can almost see the uncertainty forming as they mentally sort through everything they've just heard.

But then comes the answer. "Yeah, doc."

And that's it. The visit wraps up, and the patient leaves. From every visible angle, the appointments appears to have been successful. You communicated clearly. The diagnosis was explained. A treatment plan was delivered. The appointment moved efficiently, and another patient is already waiting in the next room.

But somewhere between the exam room and the patient's front door, it all begins to break down. Maybe the prescription is never filled because the patient misunderstood how important it was. Maybe they forgot the dosage instructions the moment they stepped into the parking lot. Perhaps the follow-up appointment is never scheduled. The dietary changes you carefully explained feel overwhelming, so nothing changes in their meals.

Days turn into weeks. Then eventually, the patient returns. What you discover is that their condition has not improved. The treatment plan was never fully implemented, and you find yourself having the same conversation all over again, retracing the exact steps you thought had already been covered.

The problem wasn't the medicine or the diagnoses. The problem was that practical knowledge about the condition and treatment never fully transferred to their daily life.

As physicians, we often assume communication happened simply because information was delivered. We explained the condition and gave careful instructions. Then we answered all of their questions. We checked every box, but true understanding is far more fragile than we often realize. In medicine, the distance between hearing information and knowing what it means can be the difference between successful treatment and preventable failure.

This pattern plays out every day in exam rooms all across the country, but why does it happen? The patient said, "Yeah, doc," so why did nothing change? Clearly, there is a disconnect happening somewhere.

EXPLANATION VERSUS COMPREHENSION

Consider the fact that the word doctor comes from the Latin word *docēre*, which actually means "to teach." It was the original job description. Long before electronic records or productivity metrics, doctors were seen as people whose job was to help people truly know what was happening inside their bodies and what to do about it.

That responsibility has not gone away, but in today's healthcare environment, the act of *teaching* is often overshadowed by the act of *doing*. Doctors diagnose and prescribe medication, and of course, they document everything. That's what they spend most of their time doing, and they are very good at it. At the same time, doctors today have learned how to move efficiently from one patient to the next because the system they work in rewards clarity of *action* over clarity of *understanding*.

Despite this, the original mandate remains unchanged. A doctor is still meant to teach. Patients expect us to teach them about their health. So, if patients expect it, if it's the original meaning of the term "doctor," then where is the process breaking down? Why are patients leaving appointments without clearly comprehending what happens next? Are they simply forgetting the instructions moments after hearing them? Are they becoming too overwhelmed by too much information delivered too quickly? Are they embarrassed to admit when they don't fully get it? Or has the healthcare system let them down by creating a process that offers explanation but doesn't have space to confirm patient comprehension?

When patients fail to fully implement their treatment plan, it's tempting to fall back on familiar explanations. *The patient is noncompliant. They're unmotivated. They're difficult.* Labels like these might offer a sense of closure. They certainly provide a reason that fits within the existing framework, but they're based on the assumption that the patient truly understood what was explained in the first place. After all, a patient can only be willfully noncompliant if they understand what compliance looks like.

In fact, I don't think it's the patient's fault at all. I think we have a major gap in patient care today. As I said, modern medicine is incredibly effective at documenting diagnoses with precision and recording treatments in detail. We're good at tracking outcomes across populations. Copious data flows through every part of the system, which gives us a clear picture of activity and results.

What we do *not* consistently measure is whether patients leave the visit with enough clarity to act on what they were told. Too often, we assume comprehension occurred simply because the conversation felt complete. The patient appeared engaged. From the physician's perspective, the visit appeared successful. The explanation was thorough, and all of their questions were answered.

But information *delivered* is not the same as information *retained.* A physician can explain something clearly, yet the patient may still leave uncertain about what to do next. Clearly, something is missing in our process, and it has created a disconnect.

THE HIDDEN VARIABLE IN MEDICINE

Every physician has encountered this disconnect, probably more times than they can count. It doesn't seem to matter if you explain a condition carefully, choosing words that are precise but also accessible. It doesn't seem to matter if you reinforce the key points multiple times and meticulously outline a treatment plan that is both logical and achievable. You've done all you can think to do within the framework and timeline available to you, and still, at the next visit, the same confusion returns.

Clearly, something in the conversation didn't fully convert into usable knowledge. The information remained external and never became internal. This is the hidden variable in medicine.

What we have *not* built, at least not with the same rigor, is a process to ensure that all of our careful explanations translate into actionable understanding. But a diagnosis without real practical knowledge makes patients feel uncertain. The patient knows something is wrong, but not what it means for their life. As a result, instructions are followed partially, or incorrectly, or not at all.

When I first started my solo practice, two things happened that, as I realized later, were incredibly beneficial for myself, staff, and patients.

First, I had time. I started with zero patients, which meant visits were slower and conversations were longer. I could teach without constantly watching the clock. So I could explain conditions carefully and answer questions thoroughly, and then I could create custom plans tailored to each person sitting in front of me.

Second, I had a file cabinet drawer filled with patient education materials collected over years of training. Pharmaceutical representatives dropped off pamphlets. Conferences provided stacks of teaching sheets. Specialists I trained with often created their own well-designed handouts that explained conditions, medications, and procedures in language patients could actually interpret.

In those days, there was no consistent system for patient education, so most of us pieced together our own approach from whatever tools and materials we could find. Some physicians had developed excellent educational resources, while others had almost nothing. I loved having those handouts. I used them constantly.

But as the years passed, something gradually changed in healthcare. The schedule became fuller, then it started getting overbooked. Visits grew shorter, and double bookings became common. Without fully realizing it, that drawer of handouts began opening less and less. Patient education still mattered, but the structure surrounding clinical practice gradually left less room for it.

As the years passed, pharmaceutical representatives continued bringing research articles, educational materials, and specialist-led presentations into the office. During lunch meetings, they would spend forty-five minutes, sometimes an entire hour, teaching physicians about a single medication, condition, or treatment approach. Entire industries invested significant time and resources into physician education because they understood that complex medical information takes time to learn and repetition to retain.

I often found myself thinking, *If it takes an hour for them to teach this to a physician, how can we expect a patient to fully understand it in just a few minutes?*

To make it more complicated, patients rarely arrive with a single isolated concern. More often, they come with a mix of issues, such as diabetes, hypertension, high cholesterol, migraines, anxiety, medication questions, potential side effects, lifestyle changes, and follow-up plans that all need to be addressed during the same appointment. What appears on the schedule as a single office visit is often a conversation covering multiple conditions, treatment decisions, and behavioral recommendations all at once.

And just as the appointment is ending, with your hand already reaching for the door, they suddenly turn around and say, "Oh, and before I go, doc, what do you think this rash is?"

The longer I practiced medicine, the harder the teaching side of healthcare began to feel.

So what's the solution? Somehow, doctors need to become teachers once again. Of course, that is easier said than done. Physicians certainly don't need more responsibility on their already-overflowing plates. Fortunately, that's not what I'm recommending. I don't think doctors need to become teachers in the traditional sense of standing in front of a room and delivering information. Instead, as healthcare evolves, the way we educate must evolve with it.

We simply need to make sure that what's explained to a patient isn't just heard, but actually retained and used. To do that, we must start measuring the success of a visit by what the patient can actually do afterward. When they have practical knowledge about their condition and their role in managing it, they cease to be passive recipients of care. They become active participants. When they do, in a sense, they stop being dependent on the physician's presence.

The challenge is that modern healthcare wasn't designed around this approach. It was designed for efficiency, for the rapid identification and treatment of disease. But if we're going to close the gap, the role of the physician has to evolve, not by expanding the workload, but by refining the focus.

In other words, this isn't about doing more. It's about doing what matters most. And that brings us back to where the profession began: doctors as teachers who engage patients in their own well-being.

HOW MISALIGNMENT HAPPENS

Doctors aren't unwilling to teach. Far from it. The problem is the system most doctors operate in. Most physicians enter practice with a primary goal to help people and make a difference. However, because of that mindset, most physicians decide to accept insurance. It seems both logical and ethical, and it's a way to make themselves accessible to as many people as possible. The thinking is that if you are going to serve a community, you should not create barriers to entry. If someone needs care, the door should be open, and that means accepting insurance.

I know this mindset because I had it myself. For a long time, I accepted all insurance because I wanted to expand access broadly. The problem is, insurance has a way of reshaping the structure of the entire practice. It introduces constraints that begin to influence how care is delivered, often in ways that are not immediately visible.

At first, everything looks as it should. Patients come in; the physician listens carefully, evaluates concerns, makes diagnoses, and creates treatment plans. Clinically, it feels sound. But behind the scenes, problems begin to arise. Claims get delayed.

Payments are denied. Reimbursements come back lower than expected. At first, it just feels like the occasional hiccup, but eventually it becomes clear these are not isolated incidents. This is an industry-wide pattern.

What makes it confusing is that the problems with insurance have nothing to do with the quality of care. The diagnoses are appropriate, and the treatments are justified. And yet, the claims keep getting rejected.

As the physician starts digging into the details, it becomes clear that the system they are operating in follows a different set of rules, and those rules don't always align with clinical logic. A diagnosis has to be listed in a specific order to be accepted. A modifier has to be placed in exactly the right spot. Certain services can't be billed together, even when both are medically appropriate and delivered during the same visit.

It turns into a process of constantly reviewing denied claims, one after another, trying to figure out what went wrong. The charts are solid. The care is correct. The documentation is thorough. The patients were treated appropriately. But none of that seems to matter.

There comes a moment in many physicians' careers when the gap between what they know and what is required of them becomes impossible to ignore. Financial pressure soon follows. Denied claims lead to delayed revenue, and delayed revenue leads to mounting expenses. The stability of the practice starts to feel uncertain.

When I reached that point in my own career, I did the only thing that made sense: I called my father for help. I explained everything: the denials, the confusion, the frustration, the growing sense that something fundamental was off. He listened carefully without interrupting me, and when I finished, he offered me a simple piece of advice.

"Find the best medical biller you can and make her your manager."

I followed his advice.

The biller thoroughly reviewed my claims and gave me her diagnosis. The problem, she explained, wasn't the medicine but the system itself. Line by line, she walked me through the logic that governed reimbursement.

"You can't list that diagnosis first. It won't pay."

"You can't bill those services together."

"You need a modifier here."

"This patient has secondary insurance. You have to bill that separately."

It felt like learning an entirely different language. Billing logic had its own rules and consequences. My medical training had not prepared me for the environment in which I was actually practicing.

To survive, I began adapting to the realities of practicing medicine. The initial changes were small. I made some adjustments to coding and paid more attention to documentation. But over time, those changes began to influence how care itself was delivered. Conversations about payment began to happen before conversations about health. I also found myself limiting what could be addressed in a single visit, a decision driven purely by billing constraints.

Even when a patient came in with multiple concerns that could reasonably be handled together in our limited time period, I began to say, "Let's bring you back to address that."

This created more visits, which meant more copays and more time away from work for the patient. Ironically, it also reduced efficiency in a way that was difficult to justify medically, but was necessary within the insurance system.

During this same period, my practice continued to grow

because patients trusted me. When they reached out with questions and concerns between visits, I answered them as promptly as I could. I happily clarified treatment plans and helped them make decisions because, after all, that is what physicians are supposed to do.

But one day, my office manager pulled me aside and told me I could no longer respond to patients in this way. When I asked why, she explained that those interactions needed to be converted into visits. If I provided guidance without bringing the patient in, there was no way to capture revenue. From a business perspective, it was unsustainable.

So I adapted again to give the system what it demanded of me, which meant more appointments but shorter visits, with more patients scheduled each day. At the same time, the documentation burden continued to grow. Notes became longer and longer as requirements became more specific. Charts followed me everywhere. I brought them home at night and worked on them at the dinner table. I sat in my car during my daughter's soccer practice, finishing documentation instead of watching her play.

This is how misalignment develops. It rarely happens all at once. Instead, it happens gradually, layer by layer, until one day you realize you're no longer practicing medicine the way you were trained. Conversations have become unsatisfyingly short, and teaching has gotten compressed into a few rushed minutes. The focus has shifted entirely toward documentation and inbox management, as the physician simply tries to keep up with the demands of the day.

And somewhere along the way, that file cabinet drawer full of patient handouts remains closed more often than open, as the materials inside slowly become outdated.

RESTORING THE STANDARD

In clinical practice today, patients often arrive at each visit with a growing backlog of concerns. They have symptoms they've been managing on their own, so the visit quickly becomes a container for everything at once, with multiple concerns, multiple symptoms, multiple treatments, and multiple decisions competing for a limited window of time.

As a result, there's rarely an extra minute to get into the underlying factors that would actually prevent disease over the long term. Education and planning get compressed or lost altogether in the time crunch.

The system itself starts to dictate what physicians prioritize. Efficiency and documentation become the priority, and throughput becomes the measure of success. The focus shifts toward what can be completed, recorded, and billed.

The results of this system are predictable. Patients leave visits with instructions, but not always with clarity or confidence. They may understand parts of the conversation without fully knowing how to apply those decisions once they return home. Between visits, they are often left to navigate the uncertainty on their own. Physicians see this every day when patients call or send messages that they don't have time to answer. They see it when a patient finally schedules a follow-up appointment after seeing a commercial or encountering a social media post about some new treatment and wondering whether it is right for them.

And when patients struggle, the system has a label for it: *noncompliance*. But that label assumes the patient knew what to do and how to do it correctly. That assumption is never tested.

If a patient doesn't fully comprehend their condition or the reasoning behind a treatment plan, every step that follows becomes uncertain. That's why patients come back with the same questions and the same confusion. Physicians find themselves repeating explanations, often in slightly different ways, hoping something will finally stick.

Somewhere along the way, despite the hard work and sincerity of doctors all across this country, medicine has lost its center. The system we've built is designed to process patients efficiently, but the original idea of the doctor as teacher is largely missing.

We need a better structure, and we don't have to add more complexity to an already complex system to get there. We just need to recognize what's been lost and restore it intentionally. Teaching must become, once again, a standard built into the way care is delivered. Until *understanding* becomes the measure of success, outcomes will continue to depend on chance instead of design.

CHAPTER 2

WHEN THE VISIT BECAME THE ENTIRE SYSTEM

"Patients do not rise to the level of information they receive. They fall to the level of systems that support them."

Imagine a college classroom on the first day of the semester. Students walk in with a sense of purpose. They carry backpacks, notebooks, binders, and pencils. They choose their seats and open their materials as they prepare themselves to learn. When the professor begins speaking, they listen carefully and take notes. The lecture lasts about fifty minutes, and it's packed with information students need to recall.

But the students know that the lecture is not the end of their learning. It is merely the starting point. After class, the real work begins. That's when students review their notes and spend time working through the material. They read, study, and test their knowledge. Concepts that seemed unclear during the lecture begin to make sense through repetition and reflection.

There is a clear structure to this process. Students receive information, then they review it and apply it. Rinse and repeat. Education isn't confined to the classroom. Every student knows that. It extends beyond class into personal study time, and that extension is what allows the knowledge shared by the professor to take root in their minds.

Now compare that with a typical doctor's visit. In many ways, it mirrors that same classroom experience. Patients wait weeks, sometimes months, for an appointment. First, they sit in the waiting room, then they move to an exam room for a more focused and important conversation.

The visit is intended to provide the patient with information about their health and recommended treatment, much like a professor's lecture. It introduces new information and sets the stage for what should happen next.

But this is where the comparison begins to break down, because while students arrive prepared to learn, patients generally do not. Most patients come to a visit without a system in place for capturing information. They don't have a notebook open on their lap or a structured way to organize what they're hearing. They aren't thinking about how they will review the material later or how they will apply it step by step. Instead, they rely on listening in the moment and remembering afterward.

That approach may work in a casual conversation. It does not work well when the information is complex or unfamiliar.

By the time the visit ends, many patients leave with little more than a memory of what was said. And memory, especially under stress, is not reliable. Medical visits often involve anxiety and unfamiliar language, and those factors make it harder for patients to process and retain information, even when they're paying close attention.

It's not surprising, then, that patients forget a significant portion of what they're told. What they do remember is often incomplete or interpreted differently than intended. Details get lost, and the overall plan can feel unclear once they're back home.

The outcomes follow a familiar pattern. Important instructions may be forgotten or partially remembered. Medications are taken incorrectly or not started at all. Follow-up steps are delayed or skipped. Patients do their best to fill in the gaps, but without a clear plan to guide them, it's hard to be consistent.

The problem is, the time between visits is where health outcomes are largely determined. That is where daily decisions are made, and treatment plans are either carried out or set aside.

A ten-to-fifteen-minute visit can introduce information and set a direction, but just like a professor's lecture, it can't create lasting understanding. That requires reinforcement and a way for patients to return to what they learned and apply it in real life.

When we expect a brief visit to do the work of an entire learning process, we set both patients and physicians up for frustration. A medical visit was never designed to carry the full weight of patient care on its own. Real outcomes are shaped by what patients know and do after the visit ends. Just as a lecture introduces material but doesn't complete a student's learning, a medical visit introduces a plan but doesn't complete the care.

WHY KNOWLEDGE BREAKS DOWN AFTER THE VISIT

Physicians put a lot of thought into every patient encounter. Behind every decision are years of training and experience. Symptoms are evaluated, risks are weighed, diagnoses are considered, and treatment plans are carefully constructed. In many cases, the work begins long before the patient even enters the room, as physicians review outside records, specialist notes, laboratory data, imaging studies, and faxed medical documents to prepare for the encounter in advance.

Yet the effort invested in creating the plan is rarely matched by a structure dedicated to helping patients carry it out afterward. Even patients who are motivated and eager to learn are often left relying on their memory alone once the visit ends.

In education, students are expected to study between classes. That expectation is built into the educational system. They are provided with homework, textbooks, maybe study guides or other materials to take with them. In healthcare, we expect patients to manage their health between visits, but we rarely provide a clear way to do that. We give instructions, but we don't always provide a framework that helps those instructions turn into consistent action.

Unfortunately, patients are often receiving important information at a time when they are least prepared to absorb it. They may be anxious about their symptoms or trying to process a new diagnosis. Their attention is divided, and their emotional state makes it harder to take in and organize new information.

Even when explanations are clear, the environment works against retention. Time is limited, and decisions must be made quickly. Once the visit ends, there is no built-in system for reviewing what was discussed and no consistent reinforcement to keep the patient on track.

The visit becomes a moment in time. It may be meaningful, but it is still only a moment. And that's simply not enough. The visit is only the starting point. What follows is what determines whether the care actually works.

CARE CONTINUES AFTER THE VISIT

Most people in healthcare are aware of this problem, but they typically see the problem as primarily about a lack of time. "If doctors just had a little more time, then they could *really* explain things to the patient." It's true, as we've said, that visits often feel rushed because schedules are packed tight these days, and physicians are asked to do more in less time. That pressure is a real issue, and it does affect the experience of care. However, the time crunch is only one part of the story.

The bigger issue is what happens outside of the clinic. It's about what happens at home, at work, within the flow of daily life. That is where medicine either works or begins to break down.

Once a patient leaves the clinic, their environment changes completely. The physician is no longer present to guide their decisions or answer any questions, and busy doctors have a hard time responding to emails or text messages in a timely manner. All that remains is the patient's memory and understanding of what was discussed, which becomes the only guide they have as they move through their day.

This is where the traditional model shows its limits. It assumes that patients can recall and interpret instructions clearly and apply them consistently in real life. Without structure to support that process, however, the assumption often falls short.

A different approach is needed, one that doesn't replace the visit but builds on it, something that can act as a bridge between the appointment and the patient's regular life. Instead of treating the visit as the entire act of care, we must begin to see it as the starting point of a larger system of treatment. In that system, patients are prepared before they arrive and then deep knowledge is developed during the visit. Then it's reinforced afterward in a way that supports daily action. Instead of relying on memory alone, patients are given tools that help them make sense of their condition and their plan, and apply it consistently.

THE SILENT EPIDEMIC OF POOR COMPREHENSION

There are few moments in medicine more discouraging than leaving an exam room with the realization that the patient didn't fully understand what you just explained to them, yet there's little the physician can do. You can't follow the patient home and trail them throughout the day. As a physician working with a tightly packed schedule and a waiting room full of patients, you must move immediately to the next visit.

At the same time, physicians know, even subconsciously, that if the patient struggles afterward, much of that unresolved confusion will eventually return through portal messages, urgent phone calls, frustrated walk-ins at the front desk, or a lot of confusion and questions during the follow-up appointment weeks later.

I remember one particular patient who brought this problem into sharp focus for me. He walked into my office carrying a stack of medical papers so large it looked like a textbook. As soon as he sat down, he started venting his frustration about how the "other doctors" never returned his phone calls or messages and how it was nearly impossible to get through to anyone.

The stack of papers contained lab results from multiple facilities, imaging reports packed with technical terminology, medication lists that were already outdated, and specialist notes that made perfect sense to the people who wrote them but very little sense to him. In many ways, it resembled the standard hospital discharge packet: an overwhelming pile of information handed to a patient who's somehow expected to make sense of it all alone at home.

He carefully set the stack on my desk and gave me an exhausted look. For months, he had been trying to manage appointments, tests, instructions, and conflicting information from different parts of the healthcare system. As he slid the papers across the desk, he said, "Here are my records. I don't really know what any of this means."

That was the real problem. He wasn't asking for more information or longer visits. He already had more information than he could reasonably process. What he lacked was clarity about what it all meant or how it applied to his daily life.

I provided what clarity I could, but then I had to send him on his way again with his giant stack of papers. This encounter wasn't an isolated patient story. Over time, that patient's story became increasingly familiar. Eventually, it stopped feeling like the exception and started feeling like a daily occurrence. Physicians reading this know exactly what I mean because versions of this patient now walk into offices multiple times a day. Frustrated patients with too much information and not enough clarity are a routine occurrence in healthcare.

There's little point in giving a patient dozens or hundreds of pages of lab reports and data if they lack a structure for seeing how all the pieces fit together. Without that structure, even well-intentioned patients struggle to follow through. It may look like a lack of effort, when in reality the patient is struggling to figure out what to do.

Patient education alone doesn't automatically create either applicable knowledge or a concrete plan of action. Patients need a way to connect all of the relevant information into a coherent whole so they know with confidence what is happening, what they should do next, and why it matters.

The patient sitting in front of me didn't need more papers added to his stack. If anything, he needed a lot *fewer* papers that had organized all of that information into a clear, usable plan. In other words, he needed guidance he could carry into everyday life.

CHAPTER 3

THE PARADOX OF MODERN HEALTHCARE

"Every advance in medicine solves a problem. Success often creates greater demand."

According to recent studies, almost half of all physicians report symptoms of burnout, and doctors remain significantly more likely to experience burnout than many other professions.[1] But burnout alone isn't the real story, or at least not the most important one.

The deeper issue is what healthcare systems have optimized themselves to do. Over the last several decades, medicine has become extraordinarily efficient at processing information, documenting visits, managing data, and increasing patient throughput. Electronic medical records, digital portals, AI tools, automated systems, and productivity workflows were all introduced with

1 Stanford Medicine, "U.S. Physician Burnout Rates Drop yet Remain Worryingly High, Stanford Medicine-Led Study Finds," Stanford Medicine News Center, April 9, 2025, https://med.stanford.edu/news/all-news/2025/04/doctor-burnout-rates-what-they-mean.html.

good intentions. Most were designed to improve efficiency and help physicians manage increasingly complex workloads.

In many ways, they succeeded. But there is an important principle that appears throughout complex systems: When efficiency increases, demand often increases with it. Economists refer to this as Jevons Paradox, which says that an increase in the efficiency of a resource usually leads to an increase, rather than a decrease, in its total consumption. In other words, when something becomes faster and more accessible, people tend to use it more, not less.

Healthcare has followed the same pattern.

As documentation became faster, more patients were added to schedules. As portals made communication easier, message volume exploded. As AI began assisting with notes and symptom searches, more patients entered the system seeking evaluation and testing. The technology improved efficiency, but instead of creating more breathing room for physicians and patients, it has mostly created a lot more volume.

In that expansion, something was bound to slip through the cracks, and the thing that has slipped the most is patient comprehension. This is ironic because today's more efficient system delivers a lot more information than ever before. Patients leave appointments with online access to labs, imaging reports, specialist notes, educational handouts, online portals, and AI-generated explanations. Yet many still walk away confused about what their condition actually means or what they are supposed to do next.

In fact, most physicians still consider the moments when a patient truly comprehends their condition or improves because of thoughtful guidance to be among the most meaningful parts of medicine. The problem is that the structure surrounding those moments increasingly works against them.

A physician's day begins long before the first patient enters the office. Charts need to be reviewed, and test results must be checked. Messages from patients, pharmacies, specialists, and staff are already waiting, and prescription refills need approval. And, of course, insurance authorizations may delay treatment before the visit even begins.

From there, the pace only accelerates. As we said, a physician's schedule these days is generally tightly packed, but each patient arrives with their own numerous concerns, a lot of emotional stress, possibly quite a bit of outside research, internet searches, and at least a few pages of prior records. Between patient visits, endless documentation and a steady flow of messages compete for attention.

The irony of this system is difficult to ignore. Medicine has become exceptionally good at generating and distributing information while, at the very same time, leaving many patients feeling overwhelmed by it.

Many patients now leave healthcare encounters with little more than a vague memory of the conversation, access to a portal with all of their test results, and maybe even a follow-up appointment already on the calendar. And they still don't understand what comes next.

The physician's medical knowledge hasn't diminished. If anything, physicians know more than ever. Their commitment to patients hasn't changed either. What *has* changed is the environment surrounding the doctor–patient relationship.

One of my friendliest patients, whom I'll call Tim, brought this reality into stark focus for me years ago.

Tim had been with me since the earliest days of my solo practice, when my schedule was still thin and flexible, and every new patient felt significant. Back then, our visits unfolded at a much slower pace. We talked about family, work, and life in addition to whatever medical issue had brought him into the office. There was room for these kinds of conversations and questions, and plenty of time to build the kind of doctor–patient relationship that drew many of us to medicine in the first place.

Then one day, after years of seeing me, Tim sat down, looked across the exam room, and asked a rather surprising question.

"What happened?"

I hesitated, unsure what he meant.

"We used to talk," he continued. "Now it feels impossible to even get an appointment with you."

There was no anger in his voice. He wasn't complaining. If anything, he sounded disappointed, as though he were mourning something special that had been lost.

As he spoke, my mind drifted to a memory that may seem unrelated at first.

Years earlier, when P.F. Chang's was at the height of its popularity, I remember walking into one of their restaurants for dinner. The lobby was overflowing with people. Families packed the waiting area, and a crowd surrounded the hostess stand. After working my way through the congestion, I finally reached the front desk only to hear that the wait for a table was two to three hours. So we turned around and left.

Sitting with Tim, I suddenly realized my practice had undergone a similar transformation. What had once been a small, accessible office had become a schedule booked weeks in advance. Every appointment slot was filled, and double bookings had become routine. The pace accelerated year after year because that was what the economics and demands of clinical practice required.

The growth was a sign of success, but it came at a cost I hadn't fully appreciated until that moment. Without making a conscious decision, I had less time for the conversations that once defined my relationship with patients. Teaching had become more compressed, and questions had to be answered more quickly (if at all). The space for simply sitting with someone and helping them realize what was happening in their health grew smaller with every passing year.

Tim wasn't criticizing me. He was holding up a mirror, and for the first time, I could clearly see what had changed.

The modern system excels at speed, access, documentation, and measurable productivity, but it leaves very little room for one of the oldest and most important relationships in medicine: the physician as teacher and the patient as learner. Is the loss of this relationship worth the increase in efficiency, especially if it has created a gap in communication? I don't think so, and I know many physicians and patients would agree.

WHEN EFFICIENCY EXPANDED THE SYSTEM

Jevons Paradox keeps showing up again and again in healthcare. Systems have become more efficient, but they have not reduced the workload. Instead, they've expanded it for almost every single person. Every new layer of healthcare efficiency, including electronic records, digital messaging, telemedicine, AI documentation, automated scheduling, and faster communication, was introduced with the promise of saving time and reducing burden. But each improvement has also lowered barriers to access, increased patient expectations, accelerated communication cycles, and created even more demands on physicians and staff.

Instead of simplifying medicine, increased efficiency has expanded the operational complexity of the system faster than human beings could realistically absorb. And that brings us directly to the deeper problem now unfolding inside healthcare.

Physicians are built to handle complexity. They spend years learning to manage uncertainty, analyze difficult cases, make high-stakes decisions, and navigate emotionally intense situations. Complexity is part of the profession's identity. Most physicians actually find purpose in solving hard problems and helping patients through difficult moments.

What they struggle with is *sustained chaos*. Chaos is being expected to operate at a pace that leaves no room to think or take a breath. Chaos is trying to keep up with constantly shifting priorities and endless interruptions. Chaos is feeling like every task is urgent while knowing there is never enough time to do any of it as thoughtfully as you would like. Chaos is spending more energy managing the system around care than delivering the care itself.

Eventually, that environment begins to erode the very meaning of the profession. When physicians lose the ability to practice medicine in a way that aligns with their training and purpose, it eventually leads them to emotionally disconnect from the work.

And that brings us back to physician burnout, a pervasive problem that can't be solved simply by telling doctors to practice more self-care or try harder to maintain work–life balance. Those things may help temporarily, but they simply do not address the underlying problem.

Ultimately, it's a structural problem. The healthcare system we have today is designed to diagnose illness, document encounters, justify billing, and process treatment efficiently. In other words, to keep the calendar full. It does this remarkably well. Most physicians are forced to schedule appointments weeks or months in advance because they're seeing so many patients.

But this has gradually moved the center of the medical visit itself. Physicians became increasingly responsible for managing the operational side of care, while teaching, listening, having real conversations, and making sure patients truly understand things has become secondary. And when doctors are constantly pulled away from the human side of medicine, even the most committed physicians eventually begin to feel drained.

In spite of it all, many physicians still love the practice of medicine. They love helping people heal and live longer, happier lives. They love the human side of care. What they struggle with is everything that increasingly stands between them and those moments.

THE INVISIBLE WORK OF MEDICAL PRACTICE

Most people assume the hardest part of the job occurs when the patient is sitting in front of the physician. They imagine difficult diagnoses with emotionally heavy conversations, or physicians dealing with the pressure of making important medical decisions while lives hang in the balance. Those things happen, and they can certainly be challenging. However, they aren't what typically drains most physicians.

The deeper burden is everything happening around the patient. It's the endless documentation requirements and the insurance negotiations that delay care or force physicians to justify decisions they already know are medically appropriate. It's the fragmented communication spread across portals, inboxes, pharmacies, specialists, and disconnected systems that rarely talk to one another efficiently. It's the unstructured follow-up that leaves patients confused about what happens next while physicians try to manage the uncertainty from a distance.

This is the hidden work of medicine. Patients rarely see it because most of it happens outside of the exam room. Yet it consumes enormous amounts of time and emotional energy every single day. Physicians often spend hours completing tasks that are necessary for the system to function, even though those tasks don't directly help patients wrap their minds around their condition or improve their long-term outcomes.

Healthcare increasingly asks physicians to do work that supports healing *and* work that merely supports the machinery surrounding healthcare, simultaneously, often at a pace that leaves little room to think clearly. Just because the amount of ancillary work has increased doesn't mean the number of hours in the week have increased. Something has to fall by the wayside, and as we said, the one thing that tends to get crowded out is *teaching*.

Let's be clear: Most physicians would *love* to spend more time teaching patients about their health and treatment plan. They know patients make better decisions when they fully grasp what's happening. They know treatment adherence improves when patients truly grasp the reasoning behind a treatment plan rather than simply receiving instructions.

The problem is that teaching requires time, attention, structure, and mental presence. Those are exactly the things the system continuously fragments.

Every decision that moves a system forward creates tradeoffs. Something improves, but something else may weaken in the process. Progress always changes the structure around it. The challenge is recognizing what was unintentionally lost while everyone was celebrating what was gained.

During one of the busiest periods of my medical career, my family gave me an unexpected Christmas gift: a set of chess lessons. I had always loved the game and had joked for years that one day, when life finally slowed down and I finally had free time, I would become a chess master in retirement. Deep down, I knew that goal was probably about as realistic as deciding to become a professional soccer player at sixty-five. But at least chess was a pursuit of the mind, and one that wouldn't punish my joints while I practiced.

A few weeks later, I sat down for my first lesson. In the middle of reviewing a game, my instructor stopped me after I made an aggressive move on the board. I still remember her pointing at the position and saying, "Before you move forward, always look at the squares you leave behind."

At the time, I thought she was simply teaching a chess strategy, but years later, that lesson stayed with me for reasons that had nothing to do with chess. As it turns out, it's true in other areas of life as well, including healthcare.

Clinical practice has moved forward in extraordinary ways. Diagnostics became faster. Treatments became more advanced. Information became digital, searchable, measurable, and instantly accessible. Healthcare systems became larger and more connected, and almost everything became more operationally efficient.

But we didn't look carefully at the squares we left behind. Somewhere along the way, an important piece lost its place on the board and inside the system. As medicine became faster and more data-driven, more digitally connected, and more operationally efficient, that piece was gradually pushed farther into the background. The physician's role as teacher began losing space inside the system.

But it's important to clarify that no one intentionally *designed* our modern healthcare system with the goal of reducing patient comprehension or weakening patient–physician communication. The changes were made for logical reasons. Better documentation improved standardization, and electronic records improved access to information. Messaging systems increased convenience, and productivity models expanded access to care for more people.

Just like good chess moves, each move forward solved a real problem, but every move also created new demands on the physician's attention.

That is where medicine finds itself today. We're better and more efficient at so many things, yet many patients leave visits feeling uncertain and anxious about what is happening inside their own bodies or what they are supposed to do next.

It's the predictable outcome of a system that constantly competes for the physician's attention. Teaching requires focus and conversation. There must be space to slow down, organize information, answer questions, and confirm knowledge. But these things are difficult to sustain in an environment built around constant interruption and compressed time.

So what can we do? How can we move some pieces forward without neglecting the piece we leave behind? Simple: We need a structured system.

WHEN STRUCTURE REPLACES CHAOS

In almost every industry, the things that matter most are supported by systems. If a company values safety, they create safety checklists and training procedures, along with repeatable protocols. If an airline values reliability, they create systems to guide everything from maintenance to communication between crew members. If a business wants consistent customer service, they create standards that help employees deliver the same experience repeatedly, regardless of who is working that day.

Important outcomes are rarely left to memory or good intentions alone. They are supported by a structured system. Healthcare grasps this concept extremely well in many areas. Entire operational infrastructures exist to make sure these processes happen consistently and accurately.

But when it comes to helping patients execute their care between visits, the structure becomes surprisingly thin. A patient may leave the office with excellent medical advice, but once they return home, they are often left trying to translate that advice into real life on their own. There's no structured system in place to help them. They are expected to remember instructions, build new habits, manage medications correctly, monitor symptoms, navigate uncertainty, and maintain consistency over weeks, months, or years.

If we're going to help them accomplish all of this, we can't just wing it. We need to create a system that helps the patient between visits. With the right structure in place, the entire experience will begin to change for the better. Patients will arrive at appointments with a stronger baseline. Instead of starting from confusion at every appointment, the conversation will begin from a shared foundation of knowledge. Questions will become more thoughtful and specific, and discussions will be more productive.

With the right structure in place, the physician no longer has to repeatedly rebuild the same educational foundation from scratch during every visit. This has a ripple effect in other areas of their job. The inbox doesn't fill up so fast because patients stop feeling lost between visits. They know what they are working toward, why it matters, and what actions they should be taking.

Patients feel more confident and capable because the path in front of them no longer feels overwhelming. Physicians feel less trapped in endless cycles of reactive problem-solving because the system itself is helping reinforce knowledge outside the walls of the clinic.

Conversations become less about recovering from breakdowns and more about advancing toward meaningful goals. At the same time, all of that invisible work of medicine begins to diminish. Physicians spend less energy correcting preventable misunderstandings. Staff spend less time managing avoidable confusion. Patients are no longer forced to guess their way through care between appointments.

Most importantly, the physician's role begins to return to what it was always meant to be: a teacher whose work doesn't end when the visit ends because what was learned during that visit continues into the patient's daily life and carries through to the next appointment.

The question is, what should a structured system that accomplishes all of this look like? How can we keep it from adding to the complexity of an already-complex process?

CHAPTER 4

EXPLANATION IS NOT ENOUGH

"Patients with low health literacy experience worse outcomes, including poorer medication adherence, lower use of preventive care, more emergency department visits, higher hospitalization rates, and increased mortality."

To create the *right* system, we first need to be very clear about the problem we're attempting to solve, and the gap we're trying to bridge. So let's make sure we understand what we're trying to solve here. To do that, we will need to look at some hard data from trustworthy sources.

Ultimately, the problem today is that modern medicine operates on an assumption so deeply embedded in the system that most of us barely notice it anymore. If we explain something clearly, we assume the patient gets it. In many ways, it is similar to clicking "I Agree" on a software update. Information was presented and acknowledgment was given, so everyone moves on, even though very few people fully comprehend what they just accepted.

That assumption allows the healthcare system to function efficiently. But anyone who has ever taught, parented, coached, or mentored another human being knows from experience that you can explain something beautifully and still not have the other person truly grasp it. What mattered was whether they understood what we were teaching and *why*. Medicine sometimes has lost sight of this disconnect because of the relentless pace of healthcare today.

Yet every physician has encountered evidence of the comprehension gap firsthand. You explain hypertension in simple language. You describe how elevated blood pressure damages blood vessels over time, even when patients feel completely normal. You connect it to heart disease and stroke risk. The patient seems engaged throughout the conversation.

Then, at the next visit, they say something like, "I thought my blood pressure was only high when I feel stressed."

You explain cholesterol and cardiovascular risk, carefully reviewing lab values and discussing why treatment is important long before symptoms appear. Months later, the patient tells you, "I didn't think it was serious because I felt fine."

You explain insulin resistance and why being consistent with medication is important, only to later hear, "I stopped taking it because I felt better."

None of this is evidence that the patient is lazy, or stubborn, or defiant. They are just signs of incomplete knowledge. There's a comprehension gap between what was said and what was actually absorbed and applied. That gap is far wider than most healthcare systems are designed to recognize. That's why we need to put a new structure in place.

Research shows that patients forget a significant portion of the information shared during medical visits, often within hours of leaving the office. Even more concerning, much of what they do remember may be remembered incorrectly. Instructions can become distorted, timelines can become fuzzy, and priorities may blur together.

Memory is only part of the problem. Research now suggests that nearly nine out of ten adults struggle to effectively grasp and use health information when medical communication becomes complex.[2] In addition, studies consistently show that patients forget between 40 and 80 percent of what physicians tell them during clinical visits.[3] The communication gap inside healthcare is far larger than most providers realize.

Patients with low health literacy consistently experience worse outcomes, including poorer medication adherence, lower use of preventive care, more emergency department visits, higher hospitalization rates, and increased mortality.

In one Medicare cohort study, limited health literacy was associated with a 52 percent higher risk of death even after adjusting for age, socioeconomic status, and baseline health.[4]

The consequences extend directly into day-to-day care. More than half of patients with chronic disease either discontinue medications early, skip doses, or fail to follow prescribed regimens consistently, which contributes to an estimated 125,000 deaths, 10 percent of hospitalizations, and roughly $100 billion in annual healthcare costs in the United States.[5] Much of this nonadherence is linked to poor patient understanding, inade-

---

2 Centers for Disease Control and Prevention, "What Is Health Literacy?," Health Literacy, last reviewed October 16, 2024, https://www.cdc.gov/health-literacy/php/about/index.html.

3 Roy P. C. Kessels, "Patients' Memory for Medical Information," Journal of the Royal Society of Medicine 96, no. 5 (2003): 219–22, https://pmc.ncbi.nlm.nih.gov/articles/PMC539473/.

4 David W. Baker, Michael S. Wolf, Joseph Feinglass, Julie A. Thompson, Jeanine A. Gazmararian, and Jenny Huang, "Health Literacy and Mortality Among Elderly Persons," Archives of Internal Medicine 167, no. 14 (2007): 1503–9, https://doi.org/10.1001/archinte.167.14.1503.

5 Sheri D. Pruitt et al., "The Silent Epidemic of Non-Adherence—Insights from the 2024 a:care Congress," BMC Proceedings 19, suppl. 10 (2025), https://doi.org/10.1186/s12919-025-00326-4.

quate communication, and lack of involvement in treatment decisions.

The problem often becomes even more visible after hospital discharge. Recent studies consistently show that although most patients leave the hospital feeling confident they grasp their diagnosis and next steps, significant gaps remain in what they actually retain.

Many patients struggle to accurately recall medication changes, follow-up instructions, and key elements of their treatment plan within the first several days after discharge despite reporting high confidence during discharge conversations.[6]

The consequences of poor communication become even more visible during care transitions. Recent studies continue to show that heart failure patients frequently leave the hospital without fully understanding discharge instructions related to medications, symptom monitoring, follow-up care, and self-management.

Research consistently demonstrates that communication failures during discharge are associated with significantly higher thirty-day readmission rates. Medicare data further show that roughly 15 to 20 percent of patients are readmitted within thirty days of discharge, creating tens of billions of dollars in avoidable healthcare costs each year, many of which are believed to be preventable through better care coordination and clearer patient communication.[7]

---

6 Payal Parikh, Priya Jaisinghani, Srivarsha Kaloth, Anagha Konakanchi, Naveena Yanamala, and Sarang Kim, "Enhancing Patient Understanding of Hospitalization and Post-Discharge Needs: The Impact of Physician-Led Verbal Communication and Teach-Back Method," Journal of General Internal Medicine 40, no. 9 (2025): 2103–10, https://doi.org/10.1007/s11606-025-09510-w.

7 Anila Sumreen, Kainat Asmat, Gideon Victor, and Erika Sivarajan Froelicher, "Effectiveness of Discharge Education on 30-Day Readmission in Patients with Heart Failure: A Systematic Review and Meta-Analysis," Journal of Health, Wellness and Community Research 3, no. 2 (2025): e90, https://doi.org/10.61919/spg5xw45.

Outpatient care reveals the same pattern. Recent studies consistently show that a large percentage of patients leave office visits without fully comprehending important aspects of what their physician explained. Research continues to demonstrate that patients frequently misunderstand medication instructions, struggle to accurately recall treatment recommendations, and often leave encounters believing they know far more than they actually do.[8]

At the same time, physicians routinely overestimate how effectively they communicated, while much of the information delivered remains filled with technical language that many patients are not equipped to fully interpret.

We ask a lot of patients. We ask them to manage medications with precise timing and dosing schedules. We ask them to change some of their deeply ingrained habits with food, sleep, exercise, stress management, and substance use. We ask them to monitor their symptoms, recognize warning signs, interpret changes in their condition, and decide when medical attention is necessary.

And we expect them to carry out all of this based on a single conversation delivered in a stressful medical environment while they are distracted by fear, anxiety, physical discomfort, time pressure, or information overload.

The problem is that the healthcare system often treats the explanation as the finish line. A physician explains the diagnosis, the visit ends, the chart is completed, and the prescription is sent. From the system's perspective, the work is done, but for the patient, the real work is only beginning.

---

8 Aloysius Wei-Yan Chia et al., "Patient-Physician Communication of Health and Risk Information in the Management of Cardiovascular Diseases and Diabetes: A Systematic Scoping Review," BMC Medicine 23, art. 96 (2025), https://doi.org/10.1186/s12916-025-03873-x.

Even when they don't fully grasp everything, patients usually nod politely during the visit. Why do people do this? Many are embarrassed to admit they don't get it. Others believe they understood in the moment, only to realize later that they can't remember what they were supposed to do. Some leave the office with every intention of following the plan, but without the confidence or clarity needed to carry it out at home.

And that is why a diagnosis may be accurate, a treatment plan may be evidence-based, and a physician may communicate with skill and compassion, yet the outcome still falls apart afterward.

The consequences of this are impossible to ignore. What appears to be a simple communication gap in the exam room is producing real-world failures outside of it.

Consider the fact that nearly six in ten adults in the United States now live with at least one chronic disease, and four in ten manage two or more. Modern healthcare increasingly depends on patients successfully carrying out treatment plans between visits. That means taking medications correctly, monitoring symptoms, adjusting lifestyle habits, following discharge instructions, coordinating specialists, obtaining labs, and recognizing warning signs early.

Yet despite this growing complexity, studies show that limited health literacy is associated with poorer medication adherence, increased hospitalization rates, higher complication rates, and worse chronic disease outcomes. Research also suggests that nearly nine out of ten adults struggle with health information at some level, especially when instructions become complicated, stressful, or medically unfamiliar.[9]

---

9 Centers for Disease Control and Prevention, "What Is Health Literacy?," Health Literacy, last reviewed October 16, 2024, https://www.cdc.gov/health-literacy/php/about/index.html.

So, the consequences aren't theoretical. Medication nonadherence alone contributes to preventable hospitalizations, emergency room visits, disease progression, and rising healthcare costs every year.

Patients discharged from hospitals often leave with medication changes, follow-up instructions, and warning signs they are expected to manage independently at home. Those with lower levels of comprehension are significantly more vulnerable during this transition period. And yet, despite the enormous real-world stakes, patient understanding itself has rarely been structured, standardized, measured, or operationalized as part of the healthcare system.

To use our earlier example, if a teacher gave a single lecture and never checked whether students retained or applied the material, we wouldn't call that a proper education. If a coach explained a complicated play once and expected flawless execution months later without reinforcement, we wouldn't call that effective coaching. Yet medicine often expects exactly this from patients managing life-altering conditions.

But what if structured patient understanding wasn't simply part of healthcare communication, but part of the entire system surrounding patient care? What if helping patients deeply grasp their condition wasn't separate from treatment, but central to whether treatment succeeded at all?

A SYSTEM DESIGNED FOR PRACTICAL KNOWLEDGE

In most areas of life, people appreciate the importance of preparation before important meetings. Before seeing an accountant, they gather their receipts and financial records. Before meeting with an attorney, they organize timelines and documents and refresh their memory on key details. There is an unspoken understanding that preparation helps the professional do their job more effectively.

Yet healthcare developed a very different expectation. Many patients still arrive assuming they simply need to show up and "tell the doctor what hurts." In an earlier era of medicine, that may have been enough. But, as we've already established, healthcare has become far too complex for that.

Today, physicians must navigate documentation requirements, insurance rules, medication histories, prior records, imaging studies, and clinical criteria that often determine which treatments are approved. They are not only caring for patients but also translating each patient's story into the documentation that healthcare systems and insurers require, making accurate histories and organized records essential.

As medicine has become more complex, preparation has become *more* important. Increasingly, patients benefit from approaching medical visits as active participants rather than passive recipients of care.

So, let's imagine a different model of care.

Before the visit even begins, the patient is introduced to simple, clear concepts that help build a foundation for the conversation ahead. Instead of walking into the appointment overwhelmed or completely unfamiliar with the terminology, they arrive with a basic framework already forming in their mind. They may not fully grasp everything yet, but they are no longer starting from zero.

During the visit, the physician's goal is no longer limited to delivering information efficiently. Now, they can focus on confirming the patient has clarity. The conversation slows down just enough to clarify misconceptions and make sure the patient can actually connect the information to their own life and decisions.

The physician actively looks for evidence that understanding is taking root.

Then, after the visit, the process continues rather than abruptly ending. The patient leaves with a structured, practical plan that can be revisited easily outside the office. It's not a thick stack of papers that they have to wade through, but something brief and to the point. They are no longer expected to rely entirely on memory or guesswork once they return home.

Gradually, the plan itself becomes part of the structure of the encounter rather than an optional extra occasionally provided. It becomes a consistent expectation built into the system's standard of care so that every patient leaves every visit with a clear, actionable plan before they walk out the door.

As a patient grows to comprehend their own diagnosis and treatment, they move from confusion to basic awareness. That basic awareness develops into active knowledge and then confident execution. They become increasingly capable of participating meaningfully in their own care rather than remaining dependent on repeated rescue from the healthcare system.

Now that clarity is the focus, everything about medicine changes for the better. Visits become clearer and more efficient because the patient arrives with context. Decisions become more precise because confusion is identified sooner. Treatment plans are followed more consistently. Outcomes improve, but something else changes too.

Medicine begins to feel different for the physician. The work becomes less repetitive because the same foundational misunderstandings stop recycling endlessly through the system. It becomes less frustrating because patients are no longer operating in a constant state of uncertainty. The physician begins to feel more aligned with the original purpose of medicine because the relationship moves away from repeatedly pushing information outward and toward building inward clarity and confidence.

Is such a system possible? Yes. I know it is because I've created it. Let's take a look.

PART 2

THE MISSING PILLAR OF HEALTHCARE

CHAPTER 5

THE MOST IMPORTANT TIME IN MEDICINE: BETWEEN VISITS

"The brain doesn't store new information exactly as it is delivered. Instead, new information gets integrated into existing mental models. That is why two patients can hear the exact same explanation and walk away with entirely different interpretations of what they heard."

Before I explain the system I created, I want to show you how I arrived at it.

It became clear to me that patients forget far more than physicians expect. There's a sizable comprehension gap, as well. Human memory doesn't function well under stress. A medical visit is often emotionally loaded before the conversation even begins. Patients may be anxious, overwhelmed, distracted, afraid, sleep-deprived, or mentally preoccupied with work, finances, family responsibilities, or the fear of what the diagnosis might mean.

Then, during a relatively short appointment, they are expected to absorb large amounts of unfamiliar information, process medical terminology, know the risks and trade-offs, remember instructions, and make decisions that may affect their health for years. That is an enormous cognitive burden for a conversation that may last only a few minutes.

Most physicians sense this intuitively, so they try to mitigate it by repeating themselves and encouraging questions. They genuinely want patients to succeed.

But a medical visit is not a neutral learning environment. When most patients walk into an exam room, they're not relaxed and mentally prepared to absorb large amounts of information. They walk in feeling fear, uncertainty, maybe physical discomfort, and they often have many unanswered questions. Some are worried about symptoms they've been trying not to think about for weeks. Others are anxious about test results, finances, family responsibilities, or what a diagnosis might mean for their future.

The patient in the exam room isn't simply an empty vessel waiting to be filled with information. Long before the physician enters the room, the patient's mind is already busy trying to interpret symptoms, predict outcomes, and prepare emotionally for the conversation ahead.

Those emotional states create stress, and stress, in turn, changes the way the brain processes information. When human beings feel threatened or overwhelmed, the brain naturally prioritizes survival over smaller details. Memory becomes less reliable. Complex information becomes harder to organize and retain.

Even when a physician explains something clearly and thoughtfully, the patient may fail to fully encode the information in a way that allows it to be recalled later. From the physician's perspective, the explanation may feel logical, organized, and entirely clear. But from the patient's perspective, something much more complicated is happening.

Patients don't simply listen to information. They filter it. Certain words immediately grab their emotional attention. Other details vanish almost as quickly as they are spoken. Some parts of the explanation get interpreted through prior experiences, family stories, or existing beliefs about health and medicine. Familiar concepts may feel clear, while unfamiliar concepts struggle to connect to anything meaningful at all.

The brain doesn't store new information exactly as it is delivered. Instead, new information gets integrated into existing mental models. If those mental models are incomplete, oversimplified, or inaccurate, the new information often becomes reshaped to fit what the patient already believes to be true.

That is why two patients can hear the exact same explanation and walk away with entirely different interpretations of what they heard.

One patient hears: "My blood pressure is elevated, but manageable."

Another hears: "I'm probably fine unless I start feeling symptoms."

This is why the issue is often bigger than simple forgetting. What frequently happens is *distortion*. Distortion occurs when instructions become overly simplified in the patient's brain in ways that unintentionally change their meaning. Timelines blur together, and priorities get rearranged. Parts of the plan are remembered while other parts disappear.

Health literacy adds another layer to the challenge. Patients are frequently asked to interpret abstract medical concepts, percentages, probabilities, and multistep treatment plans that may feel completely foreign to them. Even highly educated people can struggle to translate clinical language into practical daily action.

A patient may know intellectually that their cholesterol is elevated, yet still stare into the refrigerator later that evening, wondering what they are actually supposed to eat differently.

Another patient may know that blood pressure medication is important, but still feel uncertain about when to take it, what side effects are normal, or why missing doses is a big deal.

WHY MEDICAL INFORMATION FAILS TO STICK

So, why does medical information so often fail to stick? It helps to think about learning as a process that occurs in three stages: (1) Exposure, (2) Encoding, and (3) Recall.

Most healthcare systems focus almost entirely on the first stage. Physicians explain the diagnosis, review recommendations, discuss medications, and provide instructions. Once the information has been delivered, the system generally assumes learning has occurred.

But *exposure* is only the beginning. Real learning depends on *encoding*. Encoding is the process by which information becomes organized inside the brain in a way that allows it to be understood, retained, and used later in real-life situations. Without strong encoding, recall tends to be inconsistent and unreliable. Information may sound familiar later, but it can't be accessed clearly enough to guide decisions and behavior.

Unfortunately, the conditions for effective encoding during most medical visits are surprisingly poor. Information is often delivered quickly, even though the concepts may be complex or completely unfamiliar. Time is limited, and the patient may already feel anxious, distracted, emotionally overwhelmed, physically uncomfortable, or worried about what the diagnosis could mean for their future.

Under those conditions, the brain changes priorities. When

stress levels rise, the brain doesn't focus naturally on nuance or long-term retention. It focuses on immediate meaning and emotional survival.

- Am I okay?
- Is this dangerous?
- What happens next?

Those are the questions the brain prioritizes first. This is why many patients leave medical visits with a general impression of the conversation while struggling to recall the specific actions needed to carry the plan forward once they get home.

They remember: "I have high cholesterol."

But they may not remember: "What should I change about dinner tonight?" "When exactly should I take this medication?" "What happens if I stop taking it after a few weeks?"

A patient cannot consistently follow a plan that was never translated into practical daily behavior. Knowing blood pressure matters is very different from knowing how to manage medications, sodium intake, exercise, follow-up appointments, and warning signs over the next several months.

This also explains why discharge paperwork often fails. Patients may leave with pages and pages of instructions and educational materials, but information without an accessible structure rarely turns into usable guidance. Dense or overly clinical instructions tend to become reference material instead of practical directions. As a result, many packets sit unopened on kitchen counters or get buried in stacks of paperwork. Even when patients review them, translating clinical language into real-world action can still feel difficult.

Most patients don't need more information. They need information that is organized, simplified, reinforced, and connected directly to action. They need guidance they can revisit after the stress of the appointment fades and real life resumes.

Information answers the question, "What is this?" Comprehension answers, "What do I do now?" Many patients leave visits with fragments of the first while still needing the second.

For years, medicine operated under the assumption that clear explanations automatically produced practical knowledge, but comprehension must be instilled through reinforcement, repetition, application, and structure.

Some systems get this better than medicine does. After all, pilots aren't certified after hearing instructions once. Athletes aren't expected to master the game after a single explanation from a coach. People in these industries realize that learning happens during *encoding* and *recall* (even if they don't use those specific terms).

Patients don't need a thicker packet of paperwork but a system that makes all of that information easy to digest and put into practice. The question is no longer, "How do we explain this better?" The better question is, "How do we make this understandable enough to carry into real life?"

Care that is not remembered cannot be followed. But when understanding is reinforced properly, the treatment plan becomes part of the patient's routines, habits, and decision-making. At that point, medicine extends beyond the clinic and into everyday life, where it was always meant to exist.

A UNIVERSAL CLOSURE PROCESS

There is no universal closure process in medicine that ensures every patient can clearly explain, in their own words:

- What condition they have.
- What the treatment plan involves.
- What symptoms or warning signs they should watch for.
- What happens next.

Instead, many visits end simply because the conversation runs out of time. The prescription has been sent, so everyone moves on to the next task. The physician has another patient waiting and the medical assistant needs to turn the room. But a surgeon doesn't assume an operation was successful without verification. A pharmacist doesn't assume medication accuracy without multiple safeguards and checks. A radiologist doesn't glance at an image once and simply hope the interpretation was correct. The system depends on verification because verification reduces errors. But when it comes to patient confidence, *assumption* became the standard.

The good news is, the comprehension gap is neither inevitable nor insurmountable. Human beings are capable of learning complex information every day when it is presented clearly and consistently, and connected to practical action. Patients don't need medical school training to manage their health successfully.

Research has shown that patients retain more information when communication is simplified, reinforced over time, paired with written guidance, and structured in a way that encourages active participation rather than passive listening.[10]

10 Jason Talevski, Anna Wong Shee, Bodil Rasmussen, Georgie Kemp, and Alison Beauchamp, "Teach-Back: A Systematic Review of Implementation and Impacts," PLOS ONE 15, no. 4 (2020): e0231350, https://doi.org/10.1371/journal.pone.0231350.

In other words, people retain more when simple written plans accompany verbal discussions. They learn more effectively when they actively participate in conversations rather than sitting quietly trying to absorb information passively. And confusion is easier to identify when physicians assess patient knowledge directly instead of assuming it occurred automatically.

We don't need to give patients *more* information. In many cases, they are already overwhelmed by the amount of information they receive. Longer explanations will only increase cognitive overload rather than improve clarity.

What we need to do is create a system that reinforces key concepts instead of mentioning them only once, while simplifying complexity without talking down to patients. We need to build a structured follow-up process that confirms comprehension before patients leave the office.

A patient who truly understands their condition is more likely to notice warning signs early and take medications correctly. When they know what success in treatment looks like, they're more likely to stay engaged when that treatment becomes frustrating or inconvenient.

The goal of a medical visit should be ensuring that information becomes transformative, shaping daily decisions, routines, habits, consistency, and ultimately, long-term outcomes.

CHAPTER 6

THE HIDDEN COST OF AN UNCLEAR TREATMENT PLAN

"If you fail to plan, you are planning to fail."

Early in my career, one of the areas I spent a great deal of time treating was migraine headaches. Because of my background in both medicine and chiropractic care, I approached migraines differently than many traditional clinics. My training included occipital nerve block procedures, therapeutic Botox treatments, musculoskeletal evaluation, and neurological assessment, which allowed me to examine migraines from several different perspectives instead of viewing them strictly as a medication problem.

As the years went on, I started noticing the same pattern over and over again. Many migraine patients had already done everything they were "supposed" to do. They had seen specialists. They had completed imaging studies. They had tried multiple medications. Some carried around years of medical records filled with referrals, treatment adjustments, and follow-up visits. Yet despite all of that effort, many still felt trapped in a cycle that continued disrupting their school, work, relationships, and everyday life.

What was often missing was a clear, personalized plan patients could actually follow once they left the office.

One patient in particular stayed with me for years afterward. He was young and intelligent, but he'd been struggling with migraines severe enough to interfere with his school and daily functioning. Like many patients, he had already tried a few different treatments, but the entire process still felt disconnected. He had recommendations and various prescriptions, and he'd made all kinds of appointments, but nobody had really tied the pieces together into a practical framework that made sense in everyday life.

So instead of focusing only on suppressing symptoms, we built an individualized care plan around how he actually lived. We gathered detailed lifestyle information and looked closely at his sleep habits, exercise patterns, stress levels, nutrition, posture, muscular tension, environmental triggers, and possible food sensitivities.

We incorporated food allergy testing, evidence-based supplements, targeted medical therapies, chiropractic and neurological principles, and practical strategies he could realistically implement day to day. We also spent time discussing how and when to properly use medications once migraine symptoms began, because the timing was often just as important as the medication itself.

The goal was no longer simply, "How do we reduce migraines?" The goal became, "How do we help this patient consistently live in a way that lowers the likelihood of migraines occurring in the first place, while also giving him a clear action plan for what to do the moment symptoms begin?"

The results were remarkable. Over time, his migraines improved substantially. But what stood out even more was how much more confident and functional he became once he finally had structure and clarity around his condition. He understood his triggers better and knew which behaviors had the biggest impact. He knew what to monitor, what to prioritize, and how to respond when warning signs started appearing.

Eventually, he began thriving again academically and personally in ways that had previously felt almost impossible while living under the constant unpredictability of chronic migraines.

The plan made all the difference. For the first time, the patient had a roadmap he could actually follow outside the clinic. Care no longer depended entirely on remembering a few rushed instructions from an office visit. He now had a system that helped guide his decisions between appointments, which is where patients spend the overwhelming majority of their lives.

THE PLAN EXISTS, JUST NOT FOR THE PATIENT

Medicine became exceptionally good at building plans for physicians, but it never truly built plans for patients.

Every day in clinics across the country, physicians complete what is commonly called the "Assessment and Plan" section of the medical record. Diagnoses are documented, medications are selected, imaging is ordered, referrals are placed, and follow-up recommendations are entered into the chart.

From the clinical perspective, the plan is fully in place, but from the patient's perspective, the experience often feels very different. Patients frequently leave the office carrying fragments of a conversation they are still trying to process. Then they return home and are expected to somehow convert all of that information into consistent daily action.

There is a major difference between telling someone what they should do and helping them successfully integrate it into how they live.

A patient managing diabetes may know they need to "eat healthier," but what does that actually mean on a busy Tuesday night with kids, work stress, limited time, and years of established habits? A patient with chronic back pain may be told to exercise more, but without structure and guidance, many do not know where to begin or how to continue safely. A patient with migraines may be given medication instructions but still not understand their triggers and warning signs, or how to respond early enough to prevent escalation.

Healthcare often overestimates what patients can realistically organize on their own after a brief office visit. Consider the patient who leaves the hospital carrying multiple pages of discharge paperwork but still turns to a family member and asks, "What exactly am I supposed to do now?" Or the patient standing in their kitchen at six o'clock in the evening trying to decide whether the dietary recommendations they heard earlier actually apply to the meal in front of them.

Those situations are not unusual. They are happening every day. And they are not isolated personal failures. They are predictable outcomes of a healthcare system that was never fully designed around patient execution. The solution must be simple enough to use consistently, but structured enough to guide decisions during stressful moments. And it must be practical enough to fit inside real life.

WHY STRUCTURE CHANGES BEHAVIOR

Several years before COVID, I decided to expand beyond traditional clinical medicine and build a wellness and metabolic health company alongside my medical practice.

Day after day, I saw people struggling with issues that medications alone could not fully solve. High blood pressure, obesity, fatigue, insulin resistance, poor sleep, chronic inflammation, low energy, and declining physical health were becoming increasingly common. Many patients genuinely wanted to improve their health, but most lacked a practical system for translating good intentions into consistent behavior.

I believed there was an opportunity to create something different. I wanted to build an environment focused on more than treating illness, but on helping patients build healthier lives before illness progressed further. So I purchased a building across the street from my clinic and began developing the idea into a dedicated wellness and weight loss center.

Since this new business would operate outside traditional insurance structures, I hired a consultant who specialized in building successful cash-based wellness programs. Early in the process, he told me something surprisingly simple but profound.

"If you want people to succeed in weight loss," he said, "they need two things. First, they need to know what success looks like. Second, they need a structured plan that shows them how to get there."

The more I thought about it, the more I realized the same principle applies throughout healthcare. Patients are often told what condition they have, but they are not always shown what success looks like or given a clear path for getting there.

He explained that patients pay a premium for structure, guidance, accountability, repetition, and a process they can engage with regularly. Then he compared it to education. A student doesn't pay college tuition simply to receive information. Students pay for an organized learning experience that guides them through progress step by step. There is structure, reinforcement, accountability, feedback, repetition, and a curriculum designed to move someone from uncertainty toward mastery.

He told me wellness programs worked the same way. Patients enroll for a period of time and are given a framework to follow, study, apply, and repeat in everyday life. When that structure exists, two things begin happening simultaneously. First, patients start seeing results, and second, they begin recognizing the value of the program itself.

At the time, the insight almost sounded too simple, but the more we built the clinic, the more I realized how powerful it actually was. Over the next several weeks, we carefully refined every aspect of the program. We built clear routines, nutritional guidance, behavioral frameworks, progress tracking, educational materials, and practical daily steps patients could repeatedly return to outside the office.

We focused heavily on making the process easy to understand and realistic to implement in normal life. Patients loved the structure, and they enthusiastically followed the plan, lost weight, and started feeling better physically and emotionally. They felt more in control of their health because they finally had something clear and actionable to follow instead of vague advice like "eat healthier" or "exercise more."

Word spread quickly. Reviews improved, and referrals increased.

TIME CREATES BETTER CARE

When I first opened my medical practice in 2008, I started with zero patients. I often joke that I simply "hung up a shingle," which led to a funny moment years later when I used that phrase around a young medical student who stared at me blankly and asked, "What's a shingle?" We both laughed, and it reminded me how quickly medicine and language continue marching on.

Over the years, the practice grew rapidly. I hired exceptional physicians who were intelligent, compassionate, thoughtful, and deeply committed to their patients. Patients trusted them because they genuinely cared.

But as the practice grew, the cost and complexity of practicing medicine inside the insurance system kept growing too. In order to sustain the practice financially, we had to see more patients. As visit volume increased, so did many of the exact problems discussed throughout this book.

The front office staff would leave for the day. The medical assistants would head home. The waiting room lights would dim down. But the physicians stayed behind, sometimes for another thirty minutes, sometimes an hour, sometimes longer, trying to finish charts, respond to portal messages, clarify medication instructions, satisfy insurance requirements, refill prescriptions, and answer patient questions.

One evening, a physician I had hired, an outstanding doctor whom patients genuinely loved, was sitting alone after clinic with her face buried in her hands and her elbows resting on the desk. She was crying while trying to work through an endless queue of messages and callbacks.

I walked into the room and sat beside her. She looked exhausted, but it wasn't simply physical exhaustion. It was a deeper emotional depletion that many physicians know intimately but rarely discuss openly.

"I'm tired," she said softly. "I'm tired of getting yelled at by the front office because patients keep calling with questions. I'm tired of insurance problems. I'm tired of feeling like no matter how hard I work, it's never enough."

She was struggling precisely because she was an excellent physician who cared deeply about her patients, and her patients knew it. They trusted her and relied on her. They kept reaching back out because they still needed guidance after the visit ended.

And in many ways, that was the real problem the healthcare system had created. When patients don't fully grasp the plan, the work doesn't end. It simply moves somewhere else.

The hidden cost of not understanding is far larger than most healthcare systems recognize. Patients suffer because they feel uncertain and unsupported. Physicians suffer because they spend enormous amounts of emotional energy trying to compensate for gaps the system never fully addressed. And the healthcare system itself suffers because confusion creates inefficiency at nearly every level.

That evening in the office, sitting beside a physician emotionally drained after another long day of messages and callbacks, became a turning point for both of us.

I told her I had been exploring alternative models of care, particularly concierge medicine and direct primary care. Concierge medicine generally involves a larger yearly membership fee and often focuses on smaller patient panels with expanded access and additional services, while direct primary care has a small monthly membership fee for primary care and usually the expanded services are included. Each model came with a limited patient panel to further enhance the doctor–patient relationship.

What appealed to me most wasn't simply the business models themselves. It was the possibility of reclaiming time. Time to teach patients instead of rushing through explanations.

Time to answer questions thoroughly before confusion had a chance to grow. Time to guide patients through behavioral changes that could realistically fit into their daily lives.

Eventually, we transitioned into a direct primary care model. Almost immediately, things began improving because the environment finally created enough room for teaching.

Conversations became deeper and less rushed. Patients asked better questions because they no longer felt pressured by the clock. Physicians were able to explain conditions more thoroughly and help patients connect medical recommendations to practical daily decisions. Care plans became more actionable because there was finally time to discuss implementation instead of simply delivering instructions.

Patients felt more supported and less confused. Communication became more proactive instead of reactive. Instead of repeatedly cleaning up misunderstandings after the fact, we had more opportunities to prevent confusion from occurring in the first place.

THE INVISIBLE REWORK

Many patients become discouraged because they sincerely believe they are doing what they were told, yet their health does not improve the way they expected. Over time, they begin losing trust in the treatment plan, the process, and sometimes even themselves. Some start feeling guilty, as though they personally failed the treatment. Others become emotionally detached and convince themselves improvement simply isn't possible for them anymore.

But in many of those situations, patients were never truly given a fair opportunity to succeed. They were given information without a structure that made the information usable in everyday life.

Over time, physicians begin spending large portions of their day repeatedly rebuilding knowledge that never fully stabilized during earlier encounters. That burden also spills directly into the daily operational routine of clinical care.

Patients contact the office asking questions that may have technically been discussed during the appointment but were never fully translated into practical understanding.

- What time should I take this medication?
- Was I supposed to stop my old medication?
- Do I need the test before the follow-up appointment?
- What did the doctor mean by "watch for symptoms"?
- Can I take these medications together?
- How serious is this side effect?
- My specialist said to ask my PCP?

This creates operational fatigue throughout the entire clinic environment.

That is why the consequences of poor comprehension eventually become systemic rather than isolated. A preventable hospitalization may begin with a misunderstood medication instruction months earlier. A worsening chronic disease may trace back to vague lifestyle recommendations that never translated into sustainable daily behavior. A complication may emerge because inconsistent execution undermined the treatment over time.

Healthcare often treats these downstream events as entirely separate problems requiring entirely new solutions. But many of them are actually delayed consequences of earlier gaps in knowledge.

The costs are distributed across time, across thousands of patients, and across every level of care delivery. One missed dose here. One delayed follow-up appointment there. One preventable complication months later. Individually, those moments may appear disconnected and relatively small. Together, they form a recognizable pattern of preventable loss (of health, time, resources, trust).

It's a loss of outcomes that may have been entirely achievable under better conditions with clarity and confidence. This is why understanding cannot remain an afterthought inside healthcare.

I have seen firsthand that when we give patients clarity and structure around their condition and their treatment plan, it transforms the whole healthcare environment. Most importantly, it improves outcomes across the board for both patients and physicians.

PART 3

A NEW STANDARD OF PATIENT CARE

CHAPTER 7

TEACHING THE CONDITION

"Patients rarely change because we explain risk factors well. They change when healthcare becomes connected to something they genuinely care about protecting."

Early in my career, I started noticing something interesting during patient visits. Some of the most meaningful moments had very little to do with lab results or medication lists. They happened during conversations that, at first glance, looked almost casual.

"How are you sleeping?"

"What do you normally eat on a typical day?"

"Do you exercise much?"

"How stressed have you been lately?"

To someone sitting in the room, it might have looked like small talk. It probably seemed like I was simply trying to make patients feel comfortable or build rapport before getting down to the "real" medical discussion.

The longer I practiced, however, the more I realized that

these questions were providing information that was every bit as important as a blood pressure reading or a laboratory value. They revealed the reality of a patient's life, and that reality often explained why some people thrived while others struggled despite receiving the same diagnosis and the same recommendations.

At first, I asked those questions mostly out of curiosity. I genuinely enjoy getting to know my patients. Medicine is about people, and helping people has always been one of the most rewarding parts of the job.

Over time, though, I began noticing a pattern. Many patients were struggling because the treatment plan didn't fit the reality of their lives. The plan might look perfect on paper, the medications might be appropriate, the nutrition recommendations might be evidence-based, but if that plan required a patient to live like a completely different person than they were today, it often failed.

I saw patients who worked two jobs and barely had time to sleep. I saw parents trying to care for young children while managing chronic health conditions of their own. I saw people dealing with financial stress or demanding schedules that left little room for idealized health plans.

Many of them knew what they were *supposed* to do. The problem was figuring out how to do it consistently within the constraints of their actual lives.

Unfortunately, this is an area of treatment that doesn't receive enough attention. A patient may need to lose weight, but do they have access to healthy food? A patient may need to exercise more, but are they working twelve-hour shifts and caring for family members at home? A patient may need better sleep, but are they dealing with chronic stress that keeps their mind racing every night?

The more I paid attention, the more I realized that successful healthcare requires understanding both the disease and the person living with it. Two patients can have identical diagnoses and receive identical recommendations, yet experience very different outcomes because their circumstances, habits, motivations, and obstacles are different.

Once I understood that, my conversations with patients began to change. Instead of asking lifestyle questions casually, I started asking them intentionally. I wanted to know how they actually lived. What motivated them? What barriers kept getting in the way? What routines were already working? What support systems did they have?

The answers often explained far more than any chart note ever could. As those conversations accumulated over the years, I found myself mentally organizing the information. It was clear to me that patients needed a framework that connected medical recommendations to the realities of everyday life.

Without knowing it, I was building the earliest version of what I would eventually call PENCIL.

A BETTER WAY OF THINKING ABOUT CARE

In the beginning, the acronym PENCIL stood for **Purpose**, **Exercise**, **Nutrition**, **Counseling**, and **Integrating it into Lifestyle**.

I wasn't trying to create a formal framework or a methodology that would eventually be used by other healthcare professionals. I simply needed a better way to organize what I was learning from patients every day.

The more people I cared for, the more obvious it became that health outcomes were influenced by far more than diagnoses, medications, and treatment protocols.

I needed a way to think through those patterns, so I began organizing patient conversations around those five broad categories. PENCIL became a lens through which I could get to know patients more completely.

Purpose helped uncover motivation.

Every patient wanted something, even if they had difficulty articulating it. Some wanted to see their grandchildren grow up. Some wanted enough energy to play with their kids. Others wanted to avoid the complications they had watched a parent or spouse endure. Discovering what mattered to them gave us something to build upon.

Exercise provided insight into energy levels, physical limitations, consistency patterns, confidence, and daily habits. It helped me learn how patients interacted with movement and whether the recommendations I was considering were realistic for where they were starting.

Nutrition often exposed one of the biggest disconnects in healthcare. Most patients already knew the basics. They knew vegetables were healthier than fast food. They knew excessive sugar was not helping their health. The challenge was translating that knowledge into everyday decisions while navigating busy schedules, family obligations, financial limitations, stress, and years of deeply ingrained habits.

Counseling and motivation helped identify support systems, stressors, fears, frustrations, and the obstacles that could derail a patient's progress. Two patients with identical medical conditions could have completely different outcomes based on their mindset, environment, and support network.

Integrating it into Lifestyle tied everything together while discussing sleep patterns, work schedules, family dynamics, stress levels, routines, relationships, travel demands, and countless other variables all influencing health outcomes.

What surprised me was that PENCIL wasn't just helping me gather information. It was helping me build better treatment plans.

I remember one patient in particular. We'll call him Greg.

Greg came in for his annual Medicare wellness visit, and his chart showed arthritis in both his shoulder and hip, chronic low back pain that had gradually become part of daily life, and an elevated coronary calcium score that placed him at greater long-term cardiovascular risk.

From a purely clinical perspective, the visit could have gone in a very predictable direction. We would review the numbers, talk through the various risk factors, discuss preventive screenings, and work through the usual list of recommendations designed to improve long-term health. It was the type of appointment physicians conduct every day, built around identifying problems early and helping patients make better decisions before those problems become larger.

But by this point in my career, I had started approaching these conversations differently. As we moved through the visit, I began asking questions that extended beyond the standard medical checklist. We talked about his eating habits, exercise patterns, sleep quality, daily stress, support systems, and the overall rhythms of how he was living his life.

Eventually, we reached a question I had come to believe was often more important than many of the medical questions themselves.

"What do you enjoy doing?"

I asked it casually, but Greg answered immediately.

"Golf."

He said the answer with an energy that had been absent from the conversation up to that point.

As we kept talking, I learned that golf was far more than an occasional hobby. He played several times each week, traveling regularly to play different courses. It was one of the ways he stayed connected with friends, remained physically active, and fully enjoyed this stage of his life.

The longer we talked, the more obvious it became that Greg's ability to keep golfing was deeply connected to how he imagined the years ahead. At that point, I could have approached the visit the way medicine often does in situations like this by focusing on the clinical checklist in front of us. He needed to lose weight, improve his nutrition, strengthen the muscles supporting his joints, pay closer attention to his cardiovascular risk factors, and become more consistent with preventive care.

Every one of those recommendations was medically sound, but alone, they were simply a collection of disconnected health directives that carried very little personal meaning. So instead, I connected every single recommendation to the thing he cared about most.

"Greg," I said, "if you want to keep golfing at the level you're playing now, this is what we need to do."

We talked about physical therapy to strengthen the muscles supporting his shoulder and hip so pain would interfere less with his swing. We discussed improving his nutrition to help with weight management while lowering long-term cardiovascular risk. We talked about flexibility, mobility, and reducing inflammation so he could move more comfortably both on and off the course. We addressed his elevated calcium score, the importance of protecting his heart over the long term, and why seeing a cardiologist now could help prevent much bigger problems later.

The conversation no longer felt like a physician handing out a list of obligations. It had become personal. Greg leaned forward slightly, nodded, and smiled.

"Yeah," he said. "I have to do what I have to do if I want to keep golfing."

And in that moment, I was reminded that patients rarely change because we explain risk factors well. They change when healthcare becomes connected to something they genuinely care about protecting.

The medical recommendations hadn't changed, the science hadn't changed, the treatment options hadn't changed. What changed was that the plan now had meaning. Instead of asking Greg to improve his health because his doctor told him to, we created a plan that helped him continue doing something he loved.

That was the moment I realized PENCIL was more than a framework for gathering information. It was a way of uncovering what mattered most to patients and then looping that information back into the treatment plan itself.

The patient's purpose became the starting point for motivation. The exercise, nutrition, counseling, and lifestyle discussions revealed the barriers. And the care plan connected everything together.

Without realizing it, PENCIL had become part of my daily practice. I had never received formal training on it. There was no textbook that taught it, yet it worked so consistently that I kept using it.

PENCIL transformed the questions I asked and the way I approached patient care.

The question was no longer simply, "What disease does this patient have?" It became, "What matters most to this patient, and how do we build a plan that helps them keep it?"

THE FUTURE OF HEALTHCARE BEGINS BEFORE THE VISIT

My intention in developing PENCIL was to help patients navigate one of the most complex systems in society, a system most people are never taught how to prepare for. They are expected to participate effectively without being shown how.

But patients arrive with very different levels of preparation and organization. Some feel overwhelmed and struggle to recall symptoms, medication changes, or questions they wanted to ask. Others arrive with written concerns, updated medication lists, symptom notes, and a clear sense of what they hope to accomplish.

Patients aren't starting from the same place, and the difference in preparation influences nearly every aspect of the visit, including the quality of the conversation, the questions that get asked, the decisions that are made, and what happens after the appointment ends. Yet healthcare often treats every visit as though patients arrive under identical conditions. They do not. A prepared patient and an unprepared patient can see the same physician, receive the same diagnosis and recommendations, and still leave with very different levels of clarity and confidence.

My goal was to level the playing field by making it easier for patients to arrive with the same level of preparedness. It just makes sense. Before meeting with an accountant, most people gather tax records and financial documents. Before speaking with an attorney, they organize timelines and paperwork. Before an important business meeting, people review materials, prepare questions, and clarify objectives.

Preparation helps people make better use of limited time, yet many patients still approach medical visits believing their only responsibility is to show up. I asked myself, "What if preparation became part of healthcare rather than an afterthought? What if every patient arrived with greater clarity about their symptoms, medications, goals, and questions?"

Preparation changes the starting point of a visit. In many ways, the quality of a medical visit is often influenced before the physician ever enters the room. When patients arrive at a medical visit with even a basic level of preparation, something remarkable happens. The conversation moves forward instead of constantly starting over.

A patient who arrives with an updated medication list, written questions, symptom notes, and a basic sense of the appointment's purpose starts from a very different place than someone trying to organize everything in real time.

Preparation lightens the mental load. Patients begin recognizing concepts, terminology, and goals instead of encountering everything for the first time. Confusion gives way to familiarity, allowing more attention to be devoted to learning.

The specific actions that improve a visit are surprisingly simple:

- writing down questions
- bringing medication lists
- tracking symptoms
- reviewing prior recommendations
- taking notes
- asking for clarification before leaving.

When patients adopt these habits, they move from passive listeners to active learners. And when patients engage actively, they begin organizing information as they receive it. They identify what matters most and connect recommendations to specific actions. They ask questions when something is unclear and create mental frameworks that make information easier to remember and apply.

Most importantly, they realize what they are working toward, why it matters, and what steps come next. The benefits extend far beyond having a smoother appointment.

Prepared patients also tend to recognize problems sooner. They notice changes in symptoms, identify when progress stalls, and communicate concerns before small issues become larger ones.

Preparation also improves follow-through. Patients who grasp the purpose behind a recommendation are more likely to implement it consistently because they can connect their daily actions to long-term outcomes.

Remember, healthcare happens largely outside the clinic. It happens in the daily choices people make at home, at work, in grocery stores, restaurants, and pharmacies. The success of most treatment plans depends on those moments.

When patients have the right tools, framework, and comprehension, they become better partners in their own health. The goal is not to turn patients into medical experts. It is to help them engage more effectively in a process that already depends on their participation.

REVISITING INFORMATION

This is where a simple standardized process can make a big difference. Learning becomes more durable when patients can revisit information repeatedly rather than relying on a single conversation. Every time they review the plan, connections are reinforced and right actions become more familiar. Over time, healthy behaviors become routine.

Written plans play an important role in this process. However, not all written plans are equally effective. Many after-visit summaries are filled with valuable information but are difficult for patients to use in practice. They contain dense paragraphs, medical terminology, fragmented instructions, and large amounts of detail presented all at once.

The more I thought about this challenge, the more it influenced the development of a new PENCIL framework that can be scaled across all specialties. I saw a real opportunity to create a better learning system within healthcare. I wanted a framework that combined meaningful conversation, visual organization, written reinforcement, and practical action into a structure patients could actually use in everyday life.

The objective was to make healthcare easier to grasp. Patients needed a way to convert medical knowledge into practical daily decisions. When they can do that, they are far more prepared for every visit. They ask more thoughtful questions because they understand the context surrounding their care.

Instead of wondering, "What did the doctor say?" patients begin asking, "How do I follow the plan?"

The first question focuses on remembering information. The second focuses on applying information. One is passive. The other is active. And like I said, healthcare produces better outcomes when patients move from passive recipients of information to active participants in the implementation of that information.

EASY TO READ, EASY TO GRASP

We intentionally shifted our thinking away from traditional patient education and toward carefully designed between-visit care plans written at a level most people could process quickly and comfortably. The goal was not simply to provide information. The goal was to make that information useful.

A treatment plan should not require patients to translate complex medical terminology before taking action. Most people are already managing busy schedules, family responsibilities, work demands, and countless daily decisions. Adding unnecessary complexity only creates another barrier between knowledge and implementation.

People perform better when information is clear, practical, and easy to apply. For that reason, every element of the care plan was designed with a simple objective in mind: helping patients successfully carry out the plan after they walked out the door.

After all, the true measure of a treatment plan is not how well it is explained in the exam room. The true measure is whether patients can remember it and use it in their daily lives.

As we continued refining the system, another insight emerged. Patients don't naturally follow long paragraphs. They follow structure.

One of the earliest examples came from my own family.

One afternoon, my daughter took my granddaughter to her pediatrician because of a diaper rash that had become increasingly uncomfortable and wasn't improving on its own. It was the kind of routine visit parents make every day, something relatively minor in the larger world of medicine, but important enough when you are the one responsible for caring for a child who is uncomfortable and depending entirely on you.

During the appointment, the physician examined her, explained what was causing the irritation, and walked through the treatment plan. The recommendations were clear and medically appropriate. There was nothing particularly complicated about the diagnosis, and by all accounts, the visit itself went exactly as it should have.

My daughter listened carefully, asked a few questions, and left feeling confident she understood what needed to happen next.

But a short while later, my phone rang. It was my daughter.

There was a pause before she asked a question that immediately caught my attention.

"What am I supposed to do again?"

Nothing about the appointment had been handled poorly. The pediatrician had done exactly what physicians are trained to do. The diagnosis had been explained, and instructions had been given. All of her questions had been answered. And yet, only a short time after leaving the office, much of the conversation had already begun slipping away.

I remember thinking about how familiar this pattern really was. Patients often leave appointments believing they fully grasp what was discussed, but once they return home and the conversation is no longer sitting directly in front of them, real life immediately begins competing for attention. The mental bandwidth available during the appointment quickly disappears, and information that felt clear only minutes earlier suddenly becomes difficult to retrieve.

At the time, I had been developing some of the earliest versions of what would eventually become the PENCIL care plans. I sent her one of the written diaper rash care plans I had been working on and simply asked her to read through it.

A minute later, she laughed.

"That's exactly what the doctor told me."

Nothing about the medical information had changed. The diagnosis was the same. The treatment recommendations were the same. The physician had done nothing differently. The only thing that had changed was the format in which the information was delivered.

What had been a conversation she was already struggling to reconstruct from memory had now become a clear series of practical steps she could immediately follow at home. Instead of trying to remember scattered pieces of verbal instruction, she now had something concrete she could reference whenever uncertainty surfaced.

Over the next few days, my granddaughter's diaper rash improved exactly as expected. But what I noticed wasn't the outcome itself. It was the realization that better health outcomes sometimes do not require better medicine. Sometimes they simply require helping patients get clear on what to do once they leave the room.

That experience reinforced an important lesson for me. Patients and caregivers often do not need more information. They need information organized in a way that can be understood, remembered, and applied after the visit is over.

It struck me that nothing about the medicine had changed. The diagnosis hadn't changed. The physician hadn't done anything wrong. The only thing missing was a simple, organized way to revisit the instructions after the visit.

Think about how people use recipes, travel itineraries, packing lists, or shopping lists. Most people don't want to sort through large blocks of text when they are trying to accomplish a task. They want a clear sequence of actions that simplifies decision-making. Healthcare is no different.

That realization led us to design a behavioral checklist system rather than a traditional educational handout. It turned out to be one of the most important decisions we made.

Checklists provide clarity and reduce ambiguity, which lowers mental effort and makes decisions easier.

Rather than asking patients to remember every detail of a conversation, the checklist format allowed them to focus on the behaviors most likely to influence their health.

What should I do today? What matters most right now? What should I monitor? What habits should I repeat consistently?

Those questions became much easier to answer.

Instead of serving as a document that patients glanced at once and then forgot, the plan became something they could interact with regularly. In other words, it became a practical tool rather than a passive handout. Patients could review it, track their progress, revisit priorities, and use it to guide decisions between visits.

I remember another patient in particular. We'll call her Mary.

Mary sat across from me in the exam room as we discussed a new medication I wanted to start. It was a conversation I had repeated thousands of times over the course of my career, so familiar that I could have followed it almost automatically. We talked through why I was prescribing it, what changes we hoped to see, how often she would need to take it, and a handful of practical details that would help her begin incorporating it into her routine.

As I explained the plan, I could see that Mary was paying close attention. She was engaged and clearly wanted to know what came next. But I also recognized something I had seen in countless other patients over the years. Even when people are listening carefully, there is often far more going on beneath the surface than we realize.

She was hearing new terminology she had never encountered before. She was trying to comprehend how this medication connected to a diagnosis she was still learning to process, and at the same time, she was mentally sorting through questions about side effects, timing, insurance coverage, daily routines, and all the small adjustments that come with introducing something unfamiliar into everyday life.

None of this was visible in the simple act of nodding along during conversation.

Before wrapping up the visit, I handed her a short written care plan that summarized everything we had just discussed. It laid out the medication instructions clearly and organized the next steps in a way she could reference later.

She lowered her eyes to the page and began reading quietly. A few seconds passed before she looked up.

"Thank you," she said softly.

Then she returned to the paper.

As I watched her continue reading, I noticed a subtle change. The uncertainty that had been visible in her posture seemed to fade. She sat up straighter, studying the page in front of her with quiet concentration. Just moments earlier, our conversation had required her to hold multiple unfamiliar ideas in her head at once, trying to mentally organize information as quickly as I was delivering it. Now the information was no longer moving past her. It was sitting right there in front of her in a form she could absorb on her own terms.

She kept reading for another few moments before looking up again.

"This is really helpful," she said.

A few minutes earlier, I had been giving her instructions. Now I could see her actively working through how those instructions fit into her own life. She was no longer simply listening to a physician explain a treatment plan. She was beginning to realize what that plan would actually require once she walked out the door.

As she stood to leave, she folded the paper in half and held it in her hand for a moment. Then, almost under her breath, she said, "I can do this."

It was a small comment that could have easily passed unnoticed, but I remember realizing that the visit had ended differently than most. For the first time, I was confident that information had been delivered because I could see that it had actually taken root.

As I reflected on that encounter with Mary, I realized something else had happened that day.

Like most physicians, I cared deeply about my patients long before I ever handed her that written plan. I cared when I reviewed her history. I cared when I thought through the diagnosis. I cared when I considered the treatment options and tried to determine the best path forward.

Physicians express care in ways patients often never see. We demonstrate it through preparation, attention to detail, clinical reasoning, and the responsibility we feel for helping someone improve. Yet somewhere along the way, I began to realize that much of that effort went unnoticed.

Patients could see the prescription. They could see the laboratory orders. They could see the referral. What they did not always see was the thought, concern, and intention behind those decisions.

When Mary thanked me that day, it felt different. The gratitude was not simply for a piece of paper. It was for the clarity and confidence that the plan provided. For the first time, I felt as though the care I had invested throughout the visit had been successfully carried across the gap between physician and patient.

That realization gave me an important sense of satisfaction that a job well done was complete. It reminded me that most of us entered healthcare because we wanted to help people. Not simply diagnose disease, prescribe treatment, or complete documentation, but genuinely help another human being navigate a difficult situation.

In a small but meaningful way, it reconnected me with the part of medicine that first inspired me to become a physician.

CHAPTER 8

THE SIX ELEMENTS OF AN ACTIONABLE CARE PLAN

"When information is organized into a clear framework, patients spend less energy trying to piece everything together and more energy applying what they have learned."

As the new PENCIL framework continued to evolve, I noticed something interesting. Whether we were discussing high blood pressure, diabetes, elevated cholesterol, sleep problems, obesity, heart disease, stress management, or preventive health, patients tended to ask many of the same questions.

They wanted to know what condition they had. They wanted to know why it mattered. They wanted to know what they should do next. They wanted to know whether their efforts were making a difference. And most importantly, they wanted to know what living with the condition would realistically look like.

The specific diagnosis might change, but the structure of the conversation often remained remarkably similar. That observation led to the development of six core components that could organize almost any health discussion into a predictable and patient-friendly format. And this is where PENCIL became the current version of PENCIL.

In its latest iteration, those components are:

- *Purpose*
- *Expectations*
- *Next Steps*
- *Consistency*
- *Indications*
- *Long-Term Success*

Together, they transformed medical information from a collection of facts into a practical care plan patients could actually use and follow.

PURPOSE

The first component is **Purpose**.

Before patients can successfully manage a condition, they need to understand what it is and why it deserves attention.

Many patients know the name of their diagnosis without fully realizing its significance. They know they have high blood pressure, elevated cholesterol, prediabetes, or sleep apnea, but they do not necessarily know how those conditions affect their health or why treatment matters.

As a result, recommendations can feel disconnected from daily life. *Purpose* closes that gap by giving patients clarity about what is happening inside their bodies and why action is worth taking. It creates an emotional and intellectual connection to the condition. Even when symptoms are mild or absent, patients begin seeing why the issue deserves attention.

EXPECTATIONS

Once purpose is established, the next question naturally becomes, "What happens from here?" That is where **Expectations** enter the framework.

Patients need to perceive clearly where different paths lead. What happens if the condition is ignored? What happens if treatment is followed consistently? What outcomes are realistic? What improvements can reasonably be expected? Without those answers, recommendations may feel abstract. Patients hear instructions, but they struggle to connect today's decisions with tomorrow's outcomes.

Expectations help build that bridge. When patients are aware of the likely consequences of action and inaction, it's easier to stay motivated. The path ahead becomes more visible, and visible paths are easier to follow.

NEXT STEPS

The third component is **Next Steps**.

Over time, I came to view this as one of the most important sections in the entire framework because it answers a question patients ask constantly after leaving the office: *What do I actually do now?*

This is where medical advice turns into practical action. General recommendations may sound helpful during an appointment, but vague guidance often falls apart once patients return home. Telling someone to "eat healthier" *sounds* reasonable, but it leaves countless questions unanswered. Which foods should they focus on first? What changes will have the greatest impact? What should they reduce or eliminate?

The same principle applies to medications, exercise, sleep, stress management, and virtually every other area of health. Patients need specific next actions. The more clearly the next steps are explained, the more likely they are to be implemented.

This section is also a natural place to introduce measurable feedback. Numbers can be powerful teachers. Measurements like blood pressure readings, blood sugar levels, weight trends, sleep quality, cholesterol values, and waist circumference transform invisible conditions into visible progress. This enables patients to see the connection between their behavior and their outcomes.

CONSISTENCY

The fourth component is **Consistency**. This section grew out of one of the most common misconceptions in healthcare. Many patients hope for dramatic improvement from isolated effort. They want one great week of eating, one intense exercise program, one burst of motivation, or one perfect month to solve a problem that developed over many years.

Unfortunately, most chronic health conditions don't work that way. Most important improvements are created through repetition. Better health is usually the result of small behaviors performed consistently over long periods of time, things like taking medications as prescribed, walking regularly, getting adequate sleep, managing stress, and attending follow-up appointments.

None of these actions are particularly dramatic. Their power comes from repetition. The question isn't so much, "What should I do?" as it is "What do I need to *keep* doing?"

INDICATIONS

The fifth component is **Indications**. Patients need feedback. Without feedback, it's hard to know whether progress is happening, and that's when people begin guessing. They may interpret every symptom emotionally and assume nothing is changing when improvements are actually occurring.

Indications help patients identify what to watch, what to track, and what signals matter most. For some conditions, those Indications may be laboratory values. For others, they may involve symptom improvement, energy levels, sleep quality, blood pressure readings, or changes in physical performance.

The specific Indications vary, but the purpose remains the same. Patients become active participants in observing their own health rather than passive recipients of information.

As they begin recognizing patterns, their knowledge deepens. They see how daily decisions influence long-term outcomes, and healthcare becomes less mysterious.

LONG-TERM SUCCESS

The final component is **Long-Term Success**. This section became increasingly important because many patients approach health through a short-term lens. They search for quick fixes to problems that developed over years or even decades. They hope for rapid solutions to challenges that require ongoing attention.

Yet meaningful health improvement rarely comes from short bursts of intensity. It comes from sustainable patterns. The ultimate goal is to create a way of living that can be maintained.

Interestingly, many patients find this realization liberating rather than discouraging. Once they stop chasing quick fixes, they can focus on building healthy habits that fit their real life. They stop viewing their health as a temporary project and begin seeing it as an ongoing relationship with themselves. That new perspective creates a stronger foundation for lasting change.

WHEN ALL SIX COMPONENTS COME TOGETHER

Once all six components came together, I noticed that the visits themselves changed. Patients no longer left carrying scattered fragments of conversation and hoping they could remember everything later.

They left with structure. They knew what condition they were managing, why it mattered, what actions to take, and what measurements to track. Most importantly, they could see how the condition fit into the broader picture of their lives moving forward.

Interestingly, the information itself was often not dramatically different from what had been discussed in traditional medical visits. What changed was the organization, which had a powerful effect on their comprehension. The human brain remembers structured information far more effectively than it remembers disconnected facts.

When information is organized into a clear framework, patients spend less energy trying to piece everything together and more energy applying what they have learned. And that is ultimately what the PENCIL framework was designed to accomplish by transforming patient education into a standardized care plan.

The following images show two examples of the PENCIL framework. One demonstrates how a common medical condition can be transformed into a clear, actionable care plan. The other shows how the same framework can simplify medication education. Although the content changes for each PENCIL, the structure remains the same. This consistency allows patients to learn one framework that can be applied across conditions, medications, and procedures.

Hypertriglyceridemia

PENCIL HEALTH

PATIENT COMPREHENSIVE AND BETWEEN-VISIT CARE PLAN

Hypertriglyceridemia = high triglycerides (blood fats) • **Goal:** lower triglycerides to protect my heart & pancreas • **Focus:** healthy eating and regular activity

www.pencilhealth.com

Condition

P — Purpose

- ☐ I understand triglycerides are a type of fat that circulates in my blood
- ☐ Very high triglycerides can increase my risk of heart disease and inflame my pancreas
- ☐ I know my triglyceride goal and other cholesterol goals if my doctor has given them to me
- ☐ I avoid excess sugar, alcohol, and overeating because they can quickly raise triglycerides

E — Expectations

- ☐ I understand triglycerides often improve in weeks to months with healthy habits and treatment
- ☐ I follow my treatment plan every day, even if I feel well
- ☐ I track my weight, activity, and healthy eating between visits
- ☐ I watch for patterns that raise my levels, such as alcohol, sugary drinks, or weight gain

N — Next Steps

- ☐ I limit sugar, sweets, soda, fruit juice, and refined carbohydrates like white bread and rice
- ☐ I choose vegetables, lean protein, beans, healthy fats, and high-fiber foods
- ☐ I complete fasting blood work when ordered to monitor my triglycerides and cholesterol
- ☐ I keep my follow-up appointments and work toward my target triglyceride level

C — Consistency

- ☐ I take my medications exactly as prescribed, including fish oil, fibrates, or statins
- ☐ I do not stop or change medications without talking to my healthcare team
- ☐ I work toward a healthy weight through steady daily habits rather than quick diets
- ☐ I use reminders, meal planning, or food tracking to help me stay consistent

I — Indications

- ☐ I know to follow up with future office visit for blood work to assess levels
- ☐ I report medication side effects, muscle pain, severe stomach upset, or new symptoms promptly
- ☐ I understand sudden severe abdominal pain with nausea or vomiting may be a medical emergency

L — Long-Term Success

- ☐ I aim for at least 150 minutes of moderate exercise each week
- ☐ I get enough sleep, reduce stress, and avoid tobacco products
- ☐ I limit or avoid alcohol, especially if my triglycerides are high or very high
- ☐ I stay committed to lifelong healthy habits because triglycerides can rise again

Call Office: triglycerides remain elevated despite treatment • medication side effects • new muscle pain or weakness • questions

911/ER: Severe abdominal pain • chest pain • especially with nausea or vomiting • severe chest pain • shortness of breath

This care plan complements your medical care. It does not replace medical evaluation or individualized medical advice.

PENCIL HEALTH

Metformin

PATIENT COMPREHENSIVE AND BETWEEN-VISIT CARE PLAN

Purpose: Helps lower blood sugar and improve insulin function. This care plan guides safe, consistent daily use.

www.pencilhealth.com

Medication

P Purpose

- ☐ I understand metformin helps my body use insulin more effectively
- ☐ I understand it controls blood sugar without causing low blood sugar in most people
- ☐ I take it exactly as prescribed preferably with meals
- ☐ I do not stop it without medical guidance

E Expectations

- ☐ I understand mild stomach upset can occur when starting to take this medication
- ☐ I understand diarrhea or bloating may improve over time
- ☐ I will report persistent or severe gastrointestinal symptoms
- ☐ I understand extended-release (ER) version may reduce side effects

N Next Steps & Numbers

- ☐ I know my most recent A1C & kidney function
- ☐ I know my fasting glucose range
- ☐ I complete lab monitoring when ordered
- ☐ I understand long-term use may affect vitamin B12 levels and should be monitored

C Consistency & Compliance

- ☐ I use reminders or pill organizers if helpful
- ☐ I may temporarily hold metformin during acute illness, dehydration, vomiting, severe infection
- ☐ I may temporarily hold metformin before surgical/radiological procedures requiring contrast
- ☐ If I miss a dose, I take the next dose as scheduled (I do not double up unless instructed)

I Indications

- ☐ I always tell my care team I take metformin before procedures or imaging
- ☐ I report dehydration, severe vomiting/diarrhea, or inability to keep fluids down
- ☐ I limit & discuss alcohol intake (heavy alcohol can increase risk of serious side effects)
- ☐ I report symptoms that feel unusual or concerning

L Long-Term Success

- ☐ I refill my medication before running out
- ☐ I attend my regularly scheduled follow-up visits and lab checks
- ☐ I understand metformin supports long-term metabolic health
- ☐ I keep my nutrition, movement, and sleep health consistent

Call Office: Persistent vomiting or diarrhea or abdominal pain • unusual weakness or muscle pain • new numbness or tingling

911/ER: chest pain • stroke symptoms (sudden weakness • facial droop • speech difficulty) • severe allergic reaction

This care plan complements your medical care. It does not replace medical evaluation or individualized medical advice.

One of the most rewarding developments was watching what happened after patients had been exposed to the framework for a period of time. At first, the structure existed primarily as a tool for helping patients make sense of medical information. It provided organization and a practical roadmap for what to do after the visit ended.

Over time, however, patients started anticipating the framework themselves. They began arriving with questions organized around the same categories we used during the visit. Instead of presenting a scattered collection of concerns, they often came prepared with a clearer understanding of what information was most important and how it related to their health. They wanted to know not only what condition they had, but why it mattered. They wanted to know what outcomes to expect, what actions would have the greatest impact, what measurements they should track, and how their daily habits influenced long-term results.

In many ways, they had started thinking like participants rather than observers. The framework was no longer functioning solely as a memory aid. It was helping them develop a different way of thinking about health itself.

They began viewing conditions less as isolated medical problems and more as ongoing processes they could actively influence. They became more comfortable asking questions and recognizing the connection between daily behaviors and future outcomes. As that happened, the experience changed for physicians as well.

One of the frustrations many healthcare professionals face is the feeling of repeatedly starting from the beginning. Some repetition will always be necessary. That is simply part of caring for people. Yet when patients possess a stronger framework for true knowledge, less time is spent re-creating the foundation and sorting through confusion.

Instead, more time can be devoted to problem-solving and forward progress. The conversations become more focused, more collaborative, and thus, more productive. The structure reduces ambiguity, which allows everyone involved to spend more time discussing what matters most.

PART 4

THE SYSTEM THAT CHANGES HEALTHCARE

CHAPTER 9

A NEW LANGUAGE OF MEDICINE

"Better health doesn't always require better medicine. Often, it requires a better lifestyle plan."

Every meaningful advancement in medicine eventually becomes part of a repeatable system. They may begin as simple philosophies that sound good in theory, but they eventually evolve into repeatable processes that become woven into the everyday practice of care. This is important because if something can't be repeated consistently, it can't scale, and if it can't scale, it will never become part of the healthcare infrastructure.

History gives us plenty of examples. Sterile technique was once a breakthrough idea before becoming a standard expectation in every operating room. Monitoring vital signs eventually became so fundamental that it's difficult to imagine healthcare functioning without it. Preventive screenings followed the same path, as did surgical safety checklists. In every case, what began as innovation eventually stopped being viewed as an enhancement and became part of the normal operating structure of care itself.

Patient care planning is beginning to follow that same trajectory.

Every patient, in every setting, benefits from having a clear and consistent system for turning medical guidance into everyday action. That realization is the foundation of PENCIL Health. At its core, PENCIL is far more than just another patient handout or educational document designed to deliver information. It is a care delivery framework built around helping patients move from hearing the plan to actually living the plan.

One of the most important decisions behind our approach was to create a system that was easy to use, easy to teach, and applicable to every condition, medication, and procedure. That may sound obvious, but healthcare has a long history of taking good information and presenting it in a random way that feels overwhelming to the very people it is meant to help. Even when the physician has done an excellent job explaining the plan, the patient is often left trying to reconstruct the details later.

PENCIL was built to solve that problem by creating a consistent structure that feels intuitive from the very beginning. The physician still performs the work only a physician can do. They diagnose the condition, explain what is happening, answer questions, and develop the medical strategy that will guide treatment moving forward. The role of the PENCIL Care Plan is to take those recommendations and translate them into something patients can realistically follow once they leave the office and return to everyday life.

The framework helps patients answer a handful of simple but incredibly important questions, such as: *What exactly is happening with my health? Why does this condition matter? What should I be doing every day to improve my situation? What symptoms or changes should I be paying attention to? What habits support progress? What behaviors should I avoid because they work against recovery?*

When those questions are answered consistently, patients are no longer forced to replay fragmented conversations in their minds later that evening while trying to remember what the physician said about medications, dietary changes, exercise recommendations, warning signs, or follow-up expectations. Instead, they leave with direction and a practical roadmap they can actually follow.

Patients become more confident because they're confident about what comes next. They become more organized because they have a system they can reference instead of relying on memory. They become more engaged because for the first time, the plan feels actionable rather than abstract.

The benefits extend beyond the patient as well. Follow-up visits become far more productive because patients arrive with continuity and context instead of confusion. But the clinic itself begins operating differently.

Patient portal messages become more focused because patients know what information actually matters. Communication at the front desk becomes clearer because expectations have already been established. Medical assistants reinforce care plans more consistently because everyone is working from the same framework.

In fact, the framework is designed to function anywhere healthcare happens. It can support primary care practices, specialty clinics, wellness centers, hospitals, residency programs, and eventually entire healthcare organizations looking for a more consistent way to guide patients beyond the exam room.

The language was intentionally simplified so patients could get it immediately. The checklist format was designed to make follow-through easier. The entire structure was intentionally built around how real people think, learn, remember information, and make decisions in the middle of busy everyday lives.

BUILDING SYSTEMS PEOPLE CAN ACTUALLY FOLLOW

The medical system increasingly operates as a coordinated team effort, and the quality of care often depends on how effectively everyone involved can work from the same shared understanding.

Physicians remain responsible for diagnosing conditions, making clinical decisions, and guiding treatment. Medical assistants help reinforce continuity by supporting patient follow-through and clarifying next steps. Front office teams keep communication organized and help maintain workflow across the practice. Patients themselves carry the responsibility of bringing the plan into everyday life, where habits, routines, and decisions ultimately determine outcomes.

When everyone is operating from the same structured framework, the entire experience of care begins to feel more connected. Communication improves because expectations are clearer. The patient experiences greater consistency because the same plan is being reinforced at every point of contact. The clinic functions more smoothly because everyone is on the same page about the process and their role within it.

Perhaps most importantly, achieving this doesn't require adding layers of complexity. In many ways, it accomplishes the opposite. Having a structured framework reduces uncertainty because it makes the process easier to teach, easier to implement across teams and specialities, and easier to repeat consistently over time.

That is why the long-term opportunities extend far beyond improving individual patient visits. At a much larger level, it offers healthcare systems a scalable way to strengthen one of the most historically inconsistent parts of care, which is helping patients successfully carry out the treatment plan after the appointment ends.

ESTABLISHING A SHARED LANGUAGE

Every effective system depends on a shared language. Medicine already knows this principle exceptionally well. In fact, much of healthcare functions as effectively as it does because highly standardized systems of communication allow professionals across the entire field to understand one another with remarkable precision.

There is the language of laboratory values, where a physician can look at bloodwork and immediately know what is happening inside the body. There is the language of imaging, where radiologists, surgeons, and specialists interpret scans using shared diagnostic standards. There is the language of anatomy, disease classification, treatment protocols, and procedural guidelines that allows healthcare professionals to communicate clearly regardless of their specialty or location.

A physician practicing in one state can review a patient chart created somewhere entirely different and quickly perceive the clinical picture because the structure of communication follows a common framework. That consistency allows medicine to function at an incredibly high level.

It also reduces unnecessary confusion because everyone involved is interpreting information through the same system. And it improves coordination across specialties because providers understand one another with clarity.

While medicine has become extraordinarily sophisticated at building systems that help professionals communicate effectively with each other, what has remained far less consistent is how that care gets translated to the patient. This is where a surprising amount of variation still exists.

Every physician naturally develops their own communication style over time. Some spend considerable time walking patients through every detail of a diagnosis. Others focus more heavily on medications and treatment recommendations. Some prioritize lifestyle changes, prevention strategies, or long-term risk management. Others concentrate primarily on addressing the immediate clinical issue in front of them.

None of these approaches are inherently wrong. Healthcare is complex, and every physician learns through years of experience how to communicate in ways that feel most natural to them.

The challenge is what that variability looks like from the patient's perspective. A patient may receive one explanation from a cardiologist, hear a completely different style of explanation from an endocrinologist, receive another set of instructions from a primary care physician, and then encounter an entirely new communication approach during an urgent care visit or emergency room encounter.

Even when every provider is giving accurate medical advice, the way that information is organized, explained, and reinforced can vary dramatically from one interaction to the next. Over time, that inconsistency creates friction.

Patients are left trying to organize large amounts of information that arrive in different formats, with different priorities, different terminology, and different expectations attached to each visit. The medical recommendations themselves may be completely appropriate, but the structure surrounding that information constantly changes.

Medicine has done an extraordinary job creating standardized systems that allow professionals to communicate with one another at a very high level, yet the patient experience often lacks that same level of consistency. PENCIL is designed to help close that gap as well.

It isn't designed to replace the physician's voice or eliminate the individuality that naturally exists in patient care conversations. Rather, the goal is to create a shared language and structure no matter where care is being delivered.

That consistency creates cognitive stability. When patients repeatedly encounter information organized in predictable ways, comprehension becomes easier to maintain over time. This helps explain why standardized communication matters so much in healthcare settings where complexity can easily overwhelm patients.

The medical condition may change. The specialty involved may change. The treatment plan itself may evolve dramatically over time. But the structure surrounding the information remains familiar. That familiarity changes the patient experience in ways that are often underestimated.

Patients no longer feel like they need to learn an entirely new communication style every time they walk into a different office. They begin recognizing patterns in how care itself is organized. Instead of constantly adapting to new explanations, new formats, and new ways of processing information, they begin navigating healthcare with a growing sense of confidence.

This is where the framework begins expanding naturally across the larger healthcare system. A cardiologist can use it just as effectively as a primary care physician. A dermatologist can organize care around the same structure. Wellness clinics can adopt it. Specialists across entirely different disciplines can build conversations around the same framework while still tailoring treatment to the individual patient.

And like any effective system, it does far more than improve individual processes. Over time, it changes the culture itself. Patients who repeatedly experience organized, easy-to-follow care plans begin expecting that level of clarity from their healthcare experience.

At the same time, clinics begin naturally moving toward more standardized communication practices. Teams begin recognizing the value of consistency in how those decisions are explained and reinforced after the patient leaves the office.

Communication becomes more predictable, expectations become easier to manage, and the process of reinforcing care starts feeling far more coordinated. Healthcare teams also begin functioning differently. Physicians, medical assistants, front office staff, and support teams start operating from the same shared structure, which creates better alignment across the entire patient experience.

CHAPTER 10

THE FUTURE OF MEDICINE IS CLEAR

"A single physician, a single clinic, a single team can begin changing how patients experience care almost overnight."

As we said in the beginning, healthcare has advanced tremendously over the last century through better science, better technology, better information, and remarkable therapeutic innovation, but the next great opportunity in medicine won't come from simply creating more sophisticated treatments. It will come from improving how patients understand their health and how confidently they implement that care in their everyday lives.

Medicine will continue advancing through research, innovation, technology, and better clinical interventions, but progress can't stop there. We must place equal focus on building systems that equip patients to navigate their own healthcare journey with confidence. Healthcare improves most when patients are clear about what is happening, why it matters, and how their own decisions and daily behaviors directly shape long-term outcomes. I believe that shift will define the next generation of healthcare.

The physicians who create the greatest long-term impact will recognize that delivering excellent care requires more than clinical expertise alone. Communication has become inseparable from treatment itself, and helping patients become confident about their care may prove to be one of the most meaningful forms of medicine we can offer.

For decades, healthcare has largely operated under the assumption that once care is delivered, understanding will somehow follow naturally. Physicians explain the diagnosis, provide recommendations, answer a few questions, and trust that patients will successfully carry out those instructions once they leave the office. But experience tells us otherwise. Patients often leave feeling uncertain about what comes next, and providers find themselves repeating the same conversations while outcomes suffer in ways that better medicine alone cannot solve.

These are communication problems, and communication problems require systems designed to solve them. That is precisely where PENCIL Health enters the picture.

At its core, the PENCIL approach is to create a simple, repeatable framework that helps physicians communicate in ways patients can actually remember and implement after the appointment ends. It transforms communication from something informal and inconsistent into something structured, intentional, and built directly into the standard of care itself.

More importantly, it does this without asking healthcare providers to reinvent how they practice medicine. PENCIL doesn't require massive operational change, expensive infrastructure, or dramatic workflow disruption. It simply introduces a better framework for organizing how care is explained, reinforced, and carried out by the patient after leaving the clinic.

DOCTORS WILL BECOME TEACHERS ONCE AGAIN

This changes the physician's role in an important way. The physician of the future will not simply diagnose and prescribe. The physician of the future will teach.

When teaching becomes part of the standard of care, patients begin leaving appointments with greater clarity. They follow through more consistently. Healthcare teams spend less time repeating avoidable conversations. Compliance improves, and therefore, outcomes improve. The entire care experience begins functioning more effectively because patients know how to participate in their own treatment.

Perhaps most importantly, this kind of transformation doesn't require waiting for some distant future of medicine. It can begin inside any practice willing to communicate differently. A single physician, a single clinic, a single team can begin implementing frameworks like PENCIL immediately and begin changing how patients experience care almost overnight.

At its best, medicine has always been about helping people heal, but healing has never depended solely on what happens inside the exam room. It depends on what patients comprehend, remember, and choose to do after they leave. That is the opportunity in front of healthcare now.

Sometimes the most meaningful transformation doesn't come from inventing something entirely new. Sometimes it comes from finally improving the part of medicine we have been overlooking all along: helping patients understand. That is what PENCIL was built to do.

CONCLUSION

RESTORING TEACHING TO MEDICINE

I often think back to the file cabinet drawer in my first practice. In those early years, that drawer opened constantly. It was filled with educational materials, specialist handouts, medication guides, and teaching tools to help patients. At the time, I had the one thing every young physician has before success takes it away: time. There was time to teach, time to explain things in depth, time to make sure patients left with a clear understanding of what came next.

But as the years passed, and the practice grew, my schedule became fuller. Visits became shorter as the demands of medical care expanded. Without consciously deciding to do so, I found myself opening that cabinet drawer less and less. Eventually, it mostly stayed shut. The drawer had become a symbol of the fact that patient education still mattered, but the structure of medicine left very little room for it.

What surprised me most about developing the PENCIL framework was that, in many ways, it opened that drawer again.

Not literally, of course. The materials are different now. The technology is different. Healthcare itself is different. But the purpose is remarkably similar. Once again, patients are leaving with something designed to help them grasp their condition so they can successfully navigate the time between visits and participate more confidently in their own care.

For years, I knew I cared deeply about my patients. I carefully crafted assessments, treatment plans, and recommendations. Yet too often, that care remained trapped inside the exam room. When patients began leaving with a written care plan, it felt as though the care itself was finally transferring to the patient in a tangible way. The conversation no longer ended when the visit was over. It continued into the days and weeks that followed.

WHAT YOUR PATIENTS NEED

The medical field has accomplished extraordinary things. Over the last century, medicine has transformed through scientific discovery, technological innovation, better diagnostics, more sophisticated treatments, and a growing knowledge of how the human body works. We have become remarkably skilled at identifying disease and developing increasingly effective ways to treat it.

Yet despite all of this progress, one persistent problem continues to work against the effectiveness of the entire system. Too often, patients leave medical visits without real clarity about how to carry out their care once the appointment ends.

This challenge is easy to overlook because the clinical side of medicine often functions exactly as intended. The diagnosis is accurate, the treatment plan is appropriate, the prescription is written, and the physician has done everything correctly. Yet somewhere between leaving the clinic and returning to everyday life, the plan begins to fall apart.

Instructions are forgotten, and medications are taken inconsistently. Lifestyle changes feel overwhelming, so follow-up recommendations are delayed or ignored. Patients become discouraged, and providers end up repeating the same conversations. Ultimately, outcomes suffer in ways that better medicine alone cannot solve.

The problem is not always the care itself. Very often, the problem is communication. For decades, healthcare has invested enormous effort in standardizing diagnosis, treatment protocols, documentation systems, and operational workflows. Yet patient education, arguably one of the most important parts of long-term health outcomes, has remained surprisingly inconsistent.

Patients do not simply need more information. They need information organized in ways they can see, remember, and actually apply once they return home and begin managing their health on their own. That realization is what led to the development of PENCIL.

PENCIL was built around a simple but powerful observation, that no matter the diagnosis, patients tend to ask remarkably similar questions. They want to understand what condition they have, why it matters, what they should do next, how progress should be measured, what habits matter most, and what living successfully with the condition looks like over the long term.

The framework organizes those questions into six simple components that transform scattered medical information into a practical care plan patients can actually follow.

- **Purpose** teaches patients what condition they are managing and why it deserves attention.
- **Expectations** teach patients where different choices lead and what outcomes are realistically possible.

- **Next Steps** convert medical advice into specific actions patients can begin taking immediately.
- **Consistency** reinforces that long-term health improvement is created through repeated behavior rather than short bursts of motivation.
- **Indications** provide measurable feedback so patients can observe progress and see how their actions affect outcomes.
- **Long-Term Success** helps patients shift away from quick fixes and toward sustainable habits that support lasting health.

Individually, these components may seem simple, but together, they fundamentally change how patients experience care.

When information is organized in a predictable structure, patients stop leaving visits with scattered fragments of conversation they are struggling to remember. They leave with clarity about what they are managing, what actions they need to take, what progress looks like, and how their daily choices connect directly to their long-term health.

But the experience improves for physicians as well. When patients have a framework, less time is spent revisiting basic confusion and repeating the same explanations over and over again. Conversations become more focused. Follow-up visits become more productive. Patients arrive better prepared, ask better questions, and begin thinking less like passive recipients of care and more like active participants in their own health journey.

And perhaps most importantly, PENCIL doesn't demand expensive technology or complicated new systems layered on top of already overwhelmed healthcare practices. It simply provides a better structure for one of the most overlooked parts of care: communication.

As physicians, healthcare leaders, and clinic managers, will we continue treating patient education as an informal part of care that happens inconsistently from visit to visit? Or will we begin treating communication with the same intentionality we already bring to diagnosis, treatment planning, and clinical decision-making?

The answer will largely shape the future of medicine.

Just remember, care is complete when it is understood. The most powerful thing you can do is help patients gain clarity about their treatment. That work can begin today. It is the promise of PENCIL, and that is the future of better healthcare. A future where patient education is transformed into a standardized written care plan, and every patient leaves with a written plan.

To take a closer look at PENCIL, join us on www.pencilhealth.com.

ACKNOWLEDGMENTS

I would like to acknowledge the many mentors, physicians, educators, and healthcare professionals who helped shape my career. Throughout my training and professional journey, they taught me the importance of educating patients, communicating clearly, and building trust through teaching.

Many of these mentors developed their own methods of patient education because no standardized framework existed. They created handouts, diagrams, written instructions, and educational materials in an effort to help patients better understand their conditions and treatment plans. They recognized that patient comprehension influenced outcomes, and they witnessed the appreciation, confidence, and engagement that occurred when patients left with clear guidance.

Like me, they discovered that while patient education was universally valued, there was no common system from which to draw. Each clinician was left to create their own approach, often reinventing the process independently. Their dedication to helping patients feel confident about their care helped inspire many of the ideas explored in this book and ultimately contributed to the development of the PENCIL framework.

I am also deeply grateful to the countless patients who entrusted me with their care over the years. Every question, challenge, success, setback, and conversation taught lessons that no textbook ever could. Although no individual patient is identified in these pages, their experiences helped reveal a problem that exists throughout healthcare and inspired the search for a better solution.

Most importantly, I would like to thank my family. Since the third grade, I dreamed of becoming a physician. Pursuing that dream required years of education, long hours, sacrifices, and perseverance through both successes and setbacks. My family gave me the freedom to follow that calling and supported me throughout the journey. They were the rock I relied upon during difficult times, the source of encouragement when challenges seemed overwhelming, and the foundation that made everything else possible.

Finally, thank you to everyone who believes that healthcare is more than diagnosis and treatment. True care extends beyond the visit and continues when patients know what to do next. It is my hope that the ideas presented in this book contribute to a future where every patient leaves with a clear understanding of their care and a written plan to guide them forward.

Care is not complete when instructions are given. Care is complete when a patient leaves with a care plan they can follow.

APPENDIX

THE EVIDENCE BEHIND WRITTEN CARE PLANS

The ideas presented in this book are based on years of clinical experience, but also on decades of research demonstrating the value of written patient education and tangible take-home materials.

Across a wide range of medical specialties and healthcare settings, studies consistently show that patients benefit when verbal discussions are reinforced with clear, written information they can review after leaving the office. Written care plans help transform a single conversation into an ongoing resource that patients and families can reference throughout their care.

RESEARCH HAS SHOWN THAT WRITTEN PATIENT EDUCATION AND CARE PLANS CAN:

- Improve patient satisfaction.
- Increase patient knowledge and understanding.
- Improve recall of important medical information and instructions.

- Reduce anxiety and uncertainty after healthcare visits.
- Encourage shared decision-making between patients and clinicians.
- Improve adherence to treatment recommendations.
- Improve patients' confidence in managing their health.
- Improve psychological well-being.
- Reduce pain in appropriate clinical settings.
- Improve overall health outcomes when combined with effective patient education.
- Be most effective when written information reinforces a clinician's verbal explanation.

Together, these findings support a simple principle: when patients leave with a clear written care plan, care extends beyond the clinical visit.

The PENCIL framework was created to transform these evidence-based principles into a simple, practical, and repeatable system that helps clinicians deliver consistent written care plans across every specialty, every diagnosis, every medication, and every patient visit.

KEY REFERENCES

1. Sustersic M, Gauchet A, Foote A, Bosson JL. "How Best to Use and Evaluate Patient Information Leaflets Given During a Consultation: A Systematic Review of Literature Reviews." *Health Expectations*. 2017;20(4):531–542.
2. Unnithan AS, Chidgey BA. "Pre-Visit Education on Pain Management Options Prior to the First Clinic Visit Improves Chronic Pain Patient Satisfaction with Proposed Treatment Plans." *Pain Medicine*. 2021;22(11):2566–2574.
3. Gurusamy KS, Vaughan J, Davidson BR. "Formal Edu-

cation of Patients About to Undergo Laparoscopic Cholecystectomy." Cochrane Database of Systematic Reviews. 2014;(2):CD009933.

4. Schauffler HH, Rodriguez T, Milstein A. "Health Education and Patient Satisfaction." *Journal of Family Practice.* 1996;42(1):62–68.
5. Demir F, Ozsaker E, Ilce AO. "The Quality and Suitability of Written Educational Materials for Patients." *Journal of Clinical Nursing.* 2008;17(2):259–265.
6. Shlobin NA, Clark JR, Hoffman SC, et al. "Patient Education in Neurosurgery: Part 2 of a Systematic Review." *World Neurosurgery.* 2021;147:190–201.
7. Simonsmeier BA, Flaig M, Simacek T, Schneider M. "What Sixty Years of Research Says About the Effectiveness of Patient Education on Health: A Second-Order Meta-Analysis." *Health Psychology Review.* 2022;16(3):450–474.
8. Walsh MN, Bove AA, Cross RR, et al. "ACCF 2012 Health Policy Statement on Patient-Centered Care in Cardiovascular Medicine." *Journal of the American College of Cardiology.* 2012;59(23):2125–2143.

ABOUT THE AUTHOR

DR. JOSEPH ROTELLA is a board-certified family medicine physician and doctor of chiropractic with a passion for improving the patient experience and helping people achieve better health outcomes.

Named after his great-grandfather, Joseph Anthony Anzalone, who immigrated from Italy and lived through the Great Depression, Dr. Rotella grew up hearing stories about a man whose kindness knew no limits. His grandmother often described him as the kind of person who would give away his own jacket if someone else was cold. Those stories, combined with a childhood dream of becoming a physician, helped shape a lifelong commitment to helping others whenever and however he could.

Throughout his career, Dr. Rotella observed a recurring challenge across healthcare: Most patients understood what needed to be done but often struggled with how to do it. Whether managing a chronic condition, starting a new medication, changing lifestyle habits, or recovering from an illness, patients frequently left without a clear plan to follow.

After more than two decades in clinical practice, he came to believe that one of the most overlooked gaps in modern healthcare is the lack of standardized, actionable care plans. These observations ultimately led to the development of the PENCIL framework, a structured approach that transforms patient education into practical care plans designed to guide patients between visits.

Through his clinical practice, writing, and educational initiatives, Dr. Rotella continues to advocate for a simple idea: Every patient should leave with a written care plan and the confidence to put it into action.

The Illusion of Care is his first book.

www.ingramcontent.com/pod-product-compliance
Lightning Source LLC
LaVergne TN
LVHW100147061126
851857LV00010B/279
* 9 7 8 1 5 4 4 5 5 4 0 3 7 *